'In my ideal world every mother would have Anya on speed dial! So much sound advice combined with excellent Pilates, it's just perfect for mothers, helping them regain "control" of their bodies and laying the foundations for good body use for years to come. I cannot recommend this book highly enough.'

Lynne Robinson, Director of Body Control Pilates®

ANYA HAYES

POSTNATAL PILATES

A Recovery and Strength Guide for Life

BLOOMSBURY SPORT
LONDON · OXFORD · NEW YORK · NEW DELHI · SYDNEY

BLOOMSBURY SPORT
Bloomsbury Publishing Plc
50 Bedford Square, London, WC1B 3DP, UK

BLOOMSBURY, BLOOMSBURY SPORT and the Diana logo are trademarks of Bloomsbury Publishing Plc

First published in Great Britain 2020

A catalogue record for this book is available from the British Library

Library of Congress Cataloguing-in-Publication data has been applied for

ISBN: PB: 978-1-4729-6217-1; eBook: 978-1-4729-6218-8

2 4 6 8 10 9 7 5 3 1

Designed by Susan McIntyre. Typeset in ITC New Baskerville
Printed and bound in China by Toppan Leefung Printing

Bloomsbury Publishing Plc makes every effort to ensure that the papers used in the manufacture of our books
are natural, recyclable products made from wood grown in well-managed forests. Our manufacturing processes
conform to the environmental regulations of the country of origin.

To find out more about our authors and books visit www.bloomsbury.com and sign up for our newsletters

Contents

Introduction   **To maternity and beyond!**   6

Chapter 1   **Pilates fundamentals**   30

Chapter 2   **The fourth trimester: birth to three months**   90

Chapter 3   **Caesarean recovery**   118

Chapter 4   **Building up your strength: 'nine months in,
                nine months out'**   142

Chapter 5   **Year one and beyond**   168

Acknowledgements   186

Resources   187

About the author   189

Index   190

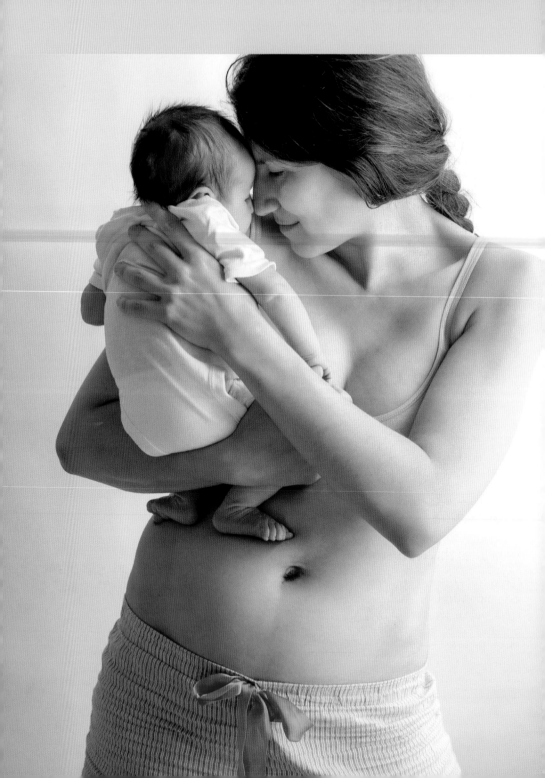

Introduction

To maternity and beyond!

Congratulations! You're a mum! Whether your baby is two weeks, two months, two years or even two decades old, this book is your toolkit of resources for postnatal rebuilding in mind, body and spirit. It aims to help you find the seat of your energies in your pelvic floor, realign your spine after pregnancy has moulded your posture for nine months and strength train your body for the daily physical graft of being a mother.

Post-pregnancy health and wellbeing: mental and physical balance

Physical and mental health are inextricably linked. It's vital that in motherhood, when our reserves are tested to the limit, we learn how to build up physical and mental resilience, so that we're able to pass this life skill on to our children. The physical depletion of pregnancy and motherhood is often overlooked and stress can very easily build up. If we're not resilient, too much stress can tip us into ill health.

Stress might be caused by the busy-ness of life, worrying about bills etc, but it's also linked to your physical environment and your diet; too much sugar or caffeine can overload your system and cause stress. Chronic stress in turn overwhelms our resilience, leading to hormonal imbalances, brain fog, fatigue and loss of physical strength. In other words, prolonged stress is detrimental to your postnatal physical healing – the healing that we assume (and hope) goes on without us paying attention to it.

How does this relate to Pilates?

If you feel *physically* weak after having babies it can have a domino effect on your emotional energy, feelings of competence, self-confidence, your sense of identity. This can spiral negatively, leading to self-doubt and self-criticism, which impacts on your health and happiness. Taking ownership of your postnatal physical recovery creates positive momentum, which can influence all other aspects of your health and wellbeing.

The intention of this book is to show you how you can replenish and renew your energy with conscious attention – how you can rebuild your reserves through bodywork, relaxation and breathing, and by putting yourself first a bit more. We're encouraged to prioritise our health during pregnancy – what you eat and drink, how much you exercise and rest – and this is deemed legitimately important because 'it's for the baby'. For some reason, though, once baby is out we feel it's no longer valid to put our health and wellbeing first. We need to reframe that.

If 'doing it for you' feels indulgent or makes you feel guilty, remember that it is still 'for the baby'. *You* need to be firing on all cylinders and in optimum health and energy, arguably more so, once your baby is out and you're tending to all their emotional, physical and snack-related needs. We also need to be happy to *be around ourselves* – you are your own constant companion. Consider how our energies transfer to the people around us. If we're stressed and depleted, this affects all our interactions. I'm definitely a nicer person to be around when I'm able to look after my body and mind. How much you move, what you eat, drink, how much you're resting – these are the building blocks of your energy. Making babies and giving birth is a huge physical feat and we need to honour the recovery.

I read recently that the average mum has approximately 17 minutes to herself every day. That probably doesn't include trips to the toilet, which are often accompanied. I *know* that your time is precious. Exercise has myriad proven benefits for body and soul: you'll feel fitter, stronger, tighter, more in control of what's happening to your body. You'll feel uplifted and energised. But, sadly, exercise can also be a source of anxiety and depletion after having a baby, if you're leaking wee when you try to run, or you're utterly exhausted and simply don't have the energy. It can become a gremlin, something that you *should* be doing.

Pilates will offer you the bridge between 'I just can't' and 'actually, I can'. Pilates can be gentle and is low impact, but deceptively challenging – if you find it too easy, you're probably not doing it right. It can also get your blood pumping and offer you that sense of achievement and a great endorphin rush without placing strain on your pelvic floor and joints. It builds your strength and vitality from the inside out: making it possible for you to begin running again without fear of embarrassing leaking, and offering you a safe way of replenishing and building vital energy on those days when an aerobic workout feels like a step too far.

What is Pilates?

Pilates is a body-conditioning method created by Joseph Pilates in the early 20th century. Pilates was a sickly child, and in his drive to put his childhood frailty behind him, he practised gymnastics, martial arts, yoga. He was a circus performer and strong man, and he drew from all these various influences to create his own exercise programme, to which he proudly attributed his physique, robust health and vitality. He was interned in the UK during World War I and during this time developed a system of exercises that wounded soldiers could perform in their beds, to help them regain strength while incapacitated. These exercises form the essence of the Pilates method and equipment today. He fled Germany before the start of World War II and set up a studio with his wife Clara in New York City, where Pilates gained popularity and prestige among dancers and boxers.

Why is Pilates so perfect postnatally?

Pilates fosters a mindful, meditative connection to your body, developing your body awareness and ability to relax. It strengthens your deep postural muscles and encourages pelvic floor awareness. Being a mum is *physically hard graft*. Pilates helps to correct your posture, which in turn reduces the strain that motherhood places on your joints.

Pilates focuses on breathing, releasing tension and strengthening the deep core muscles and pelvic floor. This will heal your body from the inside, enhancing your strength, tweaking your alignment to optimise your body's functioning. This can also help nurture a positive feeling about your body – which is particularly important if you have any sense that it has 'let you down' in your birthing or fertility experience (NB: there is *no such thing* as 'failure' when it comes to giving birth).

Tip

Classical and 'normal' Pilates classes are *not ideal for the immediate postnatal period*. There are too many potential hot spots for the abdominals and pelvic floor stress if your teacher isn't postnatal trained. So, if you're going to a class which includes classical mat Hundreds and Single/Double Leg Stretches, Roll-overs or Roll-ups, please be cautious: always keep the legs down and focus on slow conscious technique of stabilising your centre in movement – those exercises are not appropriate for your immediate postnatal recovery.

Within this book you'll find tailored Pilates exercises that you can be sure are safe and effective to rebuild strong foundations so you can get back into HIIT and running, or happily join your classical mat Pilates or gym Pilates class again soon, without worry.

The principles of Pilates

Concentration

According to Joe Pilates, Pilates requires 'complete coordination of body, mind and spirit'. So often we live on autopilot, but in a Pilates session we fully concentrate on the movement right now. Being a mum can often leave us feeling 'scatterbrained' and overwhelmed. There are too many tabs open in our brains, keeping the flotsam and jetsam of life logistics and emotional labour floating in our minds. Pilates offers an outlet to calm this chattering, being fully grounded in the present moment.

Relaxation

Motherhood is wonderful, but it's also a time of often relentless busyness and chaos, which can bring with it *completely normal* feelings of anxiety and stress. Hormonal fluctuation can contribute to a general sense of lost control and emotional instability – which only fuels our stress levels. Learning to notice your physical response to stress – how tense you are, whether you're breathing properly – is one of the most important skills to develop. Pilates encourages you to be able to recognise and switch off unwanted tension and truly relax.

Centring

Pilates movement 'flows from a strong centre'. Your 'centre' is your core muscles: the pelvic floor, deepest lower abdominals (transversus abdominis) and muscles of the spine (multifidus). Joseph Pilates noticed that he felt his spine was supported when he

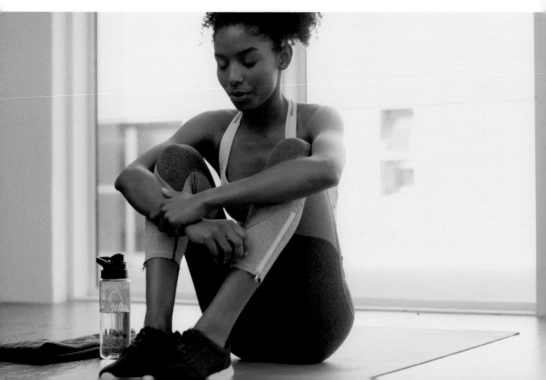

drew his tummy in tight. He used the terminology 'navel to spine' to engage the belly muscles like a corset around your waist. He called this your 'powerhouse', or 'girdle of strength'.

The 'navel to spine' terminology is now quite old-fashioned, and it can encourage you to brace the upper abdominal muscles (rectus abdominis and obliques) rather than activate your deep low strength from within. The powerhouse comes from down lower than your navel, lifting up and in. Imagine softly drawing *up* from your pubic bone and sit bones, and in from your hip bones. Imagine a diagonal line of engagement from your tailbone up towards your navel, and recruit up and in along that line.

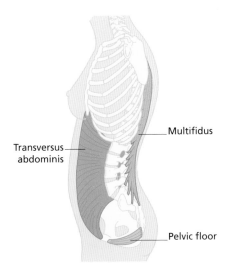

Multifidus

Transversus abdominis

Pelvic floor

Alignment

When your body is correctly aligned, your organs and muscles are balanced and optimised. Good alignment helps to reduce the impact that gravity has on your spine and joints *every day*. If your body is constantly held out of optimum alignment there's persistent strain on your body. Pilates balances your body and enables you to notice and correct your misalignments in your daily movement.

Focusing on your alignment is important not just on your mat, but also at your desk, on your commute, while you're at the playground, pushing your buggy, etc. Without good alignment, your muscles aren't balanced and optimised: your lungs won't be able to open widely to supply enough revitalising oxygen and your pelvic floor won't be able to stabilise you effectively.

Breathing

Joe Pilates said, 'Squeeze out the lungs as you would wring a wet towel dry. Soon the entire body is charged with fresh oxygen from toes to fingertips.' In Pilates, we breathe in through the nose and sigh the breath out through the mouth.

Pilates breathing is 'lateral breathing': the ribcage opens fully as you breathe in, like an umbrella opening. We breathe into the sides and back of the body rather than into the abdomen when we're moving, so that your connection to your centre can remain strong. The greatest effort in a Pilates exercise is usually performed on the exhalation, as we recruit the deep core muscles more effectively as we breathe out – *see* Piston Breath, p. 59.

Tip

Lynne Robinson at Body Control Pilates® describes your centre engagement like a dimmer switch: it should always be switched on, but there are different levels of brightness. You may need to turn it up to full brightness for more challenging work to keep you stable, but basic exercises may only need low engagement for you to feel supported.

How to breathe

Coordinated and conscious breathing is fundamental in Pilates, and it's the aspect that you might struggle with at first. Try not to worry about the breath, just remember to breathe.

Think of breath as movement: the lungs move within the ribcage during the inhalation and exhalation, like an umbrella, softly opening and closing. Visualise the diaphragm descending and widening like a big jellyfish gracefully opening as you breathe in – and feel the ribs and belly softly opening to accommodate this. And then as you breathe out, visualise the upward movement of the diaphragm lifting and drawing in.

Your lungs are located within the ribs, and the ribcage opens with your inhalation. Place your hands on your ribs. As you breathe in, feel the back and sides widening as your lungs expand. If you can feel your chest or upper shoulders rising, you're breathing too shallowly.

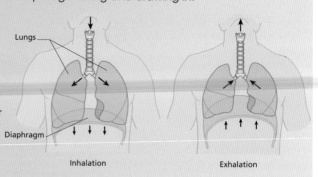

Inhalation   Exhalation

As you breathe out, feel the ribcage soften and narrow beneath your hands. Exhale with a sigh, slowly and consciously. Try to encourage your exhalation to last longer than your inhalation – try counting to five for your in-breath, and to seven with your out-breath, to expel all the air from your lungs and encourage a natural deep and full in-breath. It should feel natural and not forced.

Tip

Pilates for wellbeing

Stress is one of the biggest negative factors of modern life, and affects your physical and mental wellbeing just as much as disease. In fact, the World Health Organization predicted in 2012 that depression and anxiety would be the number-two health burden globally by 2020: bigger than heart disease, arthritis and many forms of cancer.

The breathing, mindfulness and physical challenge of Pilates has so many benefits to counterbalance stress, including:

- relaxing tense muscles and encouraging a sense of calm and wellbeing
- releasing endorphins, causing you to feel more relaxed and positive
- improving the quality of your sleep (small sleep vampires allowing), which will greatly reduce fatigue and stress.

Coordination

Coordination is a surprisingly challenging aspect of Pilates. You're training your brain to create new pathways as you repeat corrected movement patterns, overturning bad habits and locking them into our body's muscle memory. It is challenging at first, like ploughing a new trail through a field of high grass. A lot of the exercises coordinate opposite arm and leg movements, for example, which is difficult physically but also (sometimes more so!) mentally.

Flowing movements

One of the fundamental (and many) differences between Pilates and yoga is that in Pilates there is fluid, graceful movement built in to the exercise. In yoga you hold static *postures*, the movement is linking these poses together. In Pilates, the exercises are characterised by choreography, rhythm and flow.

All of these principles combine to create graceful *effortless-looking* movement. As Joe Pilates said, 'Pilates is designed to give you suppleness, natural grace and skill that will be unmistakably reflected in the way you walk, in the way you play, and in the way you work.'

Pilates exercises challenge you across all planes of movement – sitting, lying, standing, on all fours. Your muscles are worked from many different directions, which produces a very deep functional strength. It also means that it's easily transferable to your daily movements: getting up from your chair, walking up stairs, picking up your toddler, cleaning up baked beans from the floor, etc.

Stamina

There are two things you definitely need as a mum: stamina and endurance. Pilates builds stamina, both physical and mental. Endurance is developed through practising Pilates both within individual exercises – your muscles will begin to fatigue after several repetitions and your mental challenge is to not give up – and also in workouts: if your little one doesn't sabotage your session, chances are without stamina you will let yourself off the hook too easily and stop before you need to. Each time you challenge yourself just that little bit more, you're building your mind–body stamina for Pilates and for life.

Structuring your workouts

I've included workout session ideas at the end of each chapter from Chapter 2 onwards. There are many more exercises in this book than are included within these workouts, so you can create your own

> ## Tip
>
> Proper breathing benefits you in so many ways in motherhood. It's the first thing to connect you back into your nervous system to heal you after giving birth. It calms anger, softens anxiety, helps in those 'put-your-shoes-on!!' moments. It's a portable (and free!) calming tool you have with you at all times, when you're feeling tearful or exhausted. It's a cliché for a reason – taking a deep breath really does help.

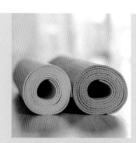

CASE STUDY

Simone, Pilates teacher and mum of two (and model in this book)

My two recoveries were vastly different. The first time, I had a third-degree tear that got infected before very slowly healing with antibiotics. The antibiotics gave me and my baby thrush and set us down a tough and painful feeding path. I had some incontinence and was super concerned it was going to stay with me. It didn't, but my trust in my body altered.

Seeing a women's health physio was one of the best things I did. Because of the third-degree tear I had been booked in for a pelvic floor test at the hospital, but had to take my baby with me, who was crying while I was examined ... far from ideal! The lady examining me said I could only hold a four-second contraction. I was horrified, especially given my profession. She referred me for a scan. In the meanwhile I saw the physio, who did an internal examination and said I was fine. The relief was huge and I could tell that as time passed I was starting to gain more strength and trust in my body.

From the start, I had been doing very gentle Pilates exercises, even if it was in bed when I had finally got Zach down. I would do some Pelvic Tilts, Knee Drops and Hip Rolls. I was always amazed that this would give me some sense of my body being my own, and slowly those connections would start firing again. Nevertheless, progress was slow. What surprised me most was that I didn't expect to walk out of the hospital still looking six months pregnant! I felt a bit cheated that my tummy hadn't just deflated! No one talks about that, how you emerge after, sore, bleeding and with a tummy. More than the look, what had been hard was that I felt like the connection to my abdominals, which had been pretty strong before pregnancy, had entirely gone. I felt like a visitor in my body and it took some work to come to terms with that.

It took a good nine months to gain a connection back to my body. That was also not something I had expected, I have danced all my life so had totally expected to naturally 'bounce back'. That was not the case at all ... it felt similar to coming back from an injury or operation, which I had done several times in my career, so in that respect I understood it and it gave me more patience, but it was frustrating.

Pilates helped my recovery in getting my body moving again. I've done Pelvic Tilts for 20 years! It makes my spine feel good and my whole body feel and work better, just Pelvic Tilts alone helped me feel better in my body. Pilates enhanced my understanding of my pelvic floor by connecting it in movement, rather than just isolating it. It also helped me to learn to release my pelvic floor in, for example, Four-point Kneeling Breathing.

My second birth was a much easier delivery and there was no tearing. I had used the EPI-NO (a pre-birth perineum trainer) while pregnant as I was really trying to avoid re-tearing – whether that was what prevented the tear or whether it would have been OK anyway I'll never know, but the recovery with no tear was significantly easier.

selection. Or just take one or two exercises and do them in isolation – if you don't have time for a 'full workout', little movement snacks throughout the day will be just as effective. I do some Spine Curls (*see* p. 82) every day, before bed or while my three-year-old climbs on me. I don't always get a chance to do much beyond that, but I always do at least that. Set yourself an accountability challenge to do *at least* two minutes/one exercise a day, and notice how you naturally *want* to grow it from there when you start feeling better for it.

Here are a few tips for planning your sessions:

- Each session should begin with some relaxation, conscious breathing and muscle release – this could be just three deep, slow breaths.
- Mobilise the spine fully if you can: flexion, lateral flexion, rotation, extension (*see* 'Movements of the spine', p. 79).
- Even doing just two exercises qualifies as a 'workout', so don't wait for the perfect time. Remember that a three-minute Pilates 'snack' is much better than nothing.

Equipment you'll need

You'll need a few things, but don't worry, nothing that involves a huge investment.

- A supportive mat – you could just do workouts on the carpeted floor but a yoga (or ideally Pilates) mat will be most comfortable and supportive for your spine.
- A stretchy band. Or you could use a scarf.
- Hand weights, of 1kg–2kg. Or, use cans of beans or full water bottles.
- A small Pilates ball. You could substitute this with a toddler football, or a cushion, depending on the exercise.

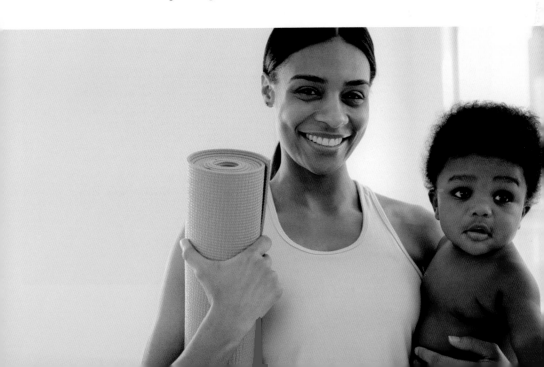

Tip

Don't wait for the 'perfect time' to do your workouts. With babies and children, the perfect moment almost never happens – and if it does, you're interrupted after three seconds. All of these exercises can be done with or around your children. Don't give up on the idea if you lose your free space. Get them involved. Make them see mummy prioritising her strength, moving and focusing time on self-care. Let them see you valuing yourself. *Build it into the mayhem* rather than waiting for the right time. Break it down into movement 'snacks' throughout the day – 10 minutes here, 3 minutes there, 30 seconds there – this is *just as valuable* as a longer workout. The more you build exercise into your life, the more you'll crave it and find more time to do it, in a positive cycle.

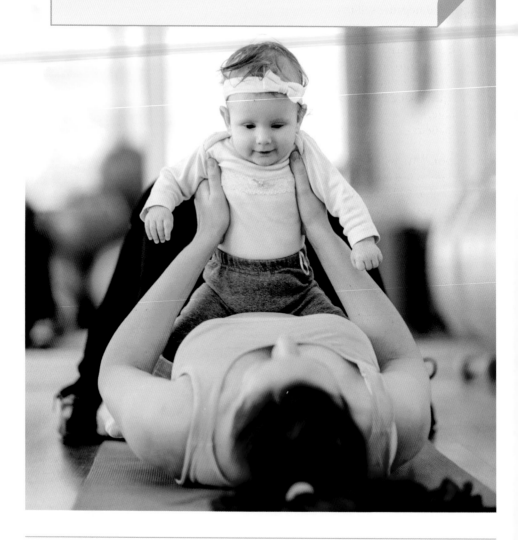

Four pillars of self-care

To get the most of your Pilates practice, aim to scaffold it with four self-care pillars for a healthy life: rest, rehydrate, refuel, revitalise!

- *Rest* – Notice I say *rest*, not sleep. Whatever stage of motherhood you're in, sleep can be emotively elusive at times, something that we can never fully control, particularly in the early days. It can be detrimental to your emotional energy to be told 'you need more sleep' as if it's something you can magically turn around, when your baby wakes every 45 minutes or your toddler thinks sleep is for losers (or maybe your six-year-old still occasionally creeps into your bed at 4am). Getting enough sleep is *such a big deal.* Lack of sleep leaves you open to heightened emotions, such as sadness, anger and negative self-talk. Lack of sleep undoubtedly puts you at higher risk of depression.

  We need to learn to incorporate rest and nervous system restoration into our days so that we can benefit fully from the sleep that we *are* getting, even if a solid eight hours is denied to us. Just taking five deep breaths regularly will help you to recharge, soothe your nervous system, calm you out of negative automatic responses.

- *Rehydrate* – We need to drink an adequate volume of water to function: to feel energised, to absorb the most nutrients from our food, to feel alert. Remember that pot plant that you always forget to water? We are all just slightly more complex pot plants, and we wilt exactly the same way when dehydrated. Coffee, sadly, is not a good hydrator, and can also block your gut absorption of valuable nutrients and minerals such as iron, so it's worth substituting your regular flat white with a simple flat H_2O to optimise your nutritional health. Caffeine can also be one of the contributing factors to pelvic floor dysfunction and urinary incontinence (*see* p. 42) – so if you're suffering, it might be worth looking at your coffee/tea/Diet Coke intake.

- *Refuel* – Mums can fall into the trap of relying on survival-mode coffee, grab-and-go food, hoovering up leftover cold fish fingers (yum!). If you're breastfeeding, the sugar lure seems to be even stronger; sleep deprivation definitely makes you lean towards the carrot cake rather than the carrot soup. Be kind to yourself. The joy of a sugar hit is *essential,* sometimes. Commit to noticing whether your diet really isn't helping you to rebuild your energy and vitality from the inside and see if you can make micro changes to move in the right direction.

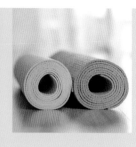

CASE STUDY

Ria, mum of one

I feel a good connection to my body through Pilates and practised throughout my pregnancy. I could pay attention to where the aches and pains were and soothe them. Having previously been taught that exercise is about punishing your body, Pilates really felt like loving it! Postnatally, when there were lots of other things I couldn't do yet, I could manage some gentle Pilates. And that was encouraging.

Gut health has a profound impact on wellbeing – around 90 per cent of serotonin, your 'happy chemical', responsible for feelings of happiness and wellbeing, is produced in your gut. Pregnancy and birth can have a huge impact on gut health. Hormones, pregnancy nausea and its effect on your appetite and digestion; caffeine; sugar; not to mention Caesarean birth and antibiotics, all influence your gut microbiome. Therefore, there's potentially a (generally unexplored) link between gut health and maternal mental health/postnatal depression. So, noticing whether your gut may be sabotaging your mood is really important. I recommend Eve Kalinik's wonderful book *Be Good to Your Gut*, and have included details in the Resources. Tummy massage is also a key tool for enhancing gut health (*see* p. 124).

- *Revitalise* – Move your body every day. I'm not talking about 'Fat-burning Baby Zumba Bootcamp HIIT' to 'lose the mum tum' and 'get your body back'. I'm talking about being curious about how your body works and what it needs in order to thrive. What makes you *feel better*. Movement might mean simply breathing adequately in the early days. It can mean massage to move your connective tissue, circulation, organs – which are still recalibrating their positions post birth. It can be walking, swimming, kitchen disco dancing… It means oxygenating your body, revitalising your tissue, your soul. It also can mean movement of your thoughts and mind through moments of mindfulness meditation or journalling, to help you when you're emotionally stuck.

Postnatal depletion

My eldest son often talks about when I 'built' him in my tummy. I love this. It makes me feel like I had some artisan craftsperson level of skill and talent in the creation of a new human. It also makes me realise the level of intense toil, materials and focus needed to build a baby – but we do this without consciously 'doing' anything, and we're keen not to be seen as 'less capable than normal' so we often ignore its huge impact. Building a baby is tough on your body. The mistake we make as a society is belittling this and expecting everyone to crack on as normal, preferably showcasing a 'spectacular post-baby body' as soon as your baby is out.

Pregnancy and childbirth are like a hormonal volcano. Apart from all the eyelashes and toes you made, you also conjured up an entirely new organ for yourself, the placenta. One that magically creates your supercharged hormone levels to sustain and nourish you and your baby throughout the nine-plus months. Your body sends all available nutrients, minerals, hydration, *everything*, to your baby, with you just getting on with normal life while this alchemy is happening. Once baby and placenta are out, there's a tremendously powerful watershed in this level of hormonal activity, when you lose the magic provided by this extra organ. It takes time for your body to negotiate this new terrain. *Of course* you don't feel 'normal' yet. Of course your body is depleted and you feel a bit discombobulated.

The sheer pace of modern motherhood means that we usually ignore symptoms of depletion, hoping they will somehow miraculously reset themselves in time. Heightened anxiety, immense

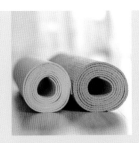

CASE STUDY

Nicola, Pilates teacher and mum of one

Your body doesn't feel like your own when you've just had a baby, and let's face it, neither does your mind! Returning to Pilates after I'd had my daughter allowed me to focus on both. It gave me time to breathe, relax and to reconnect. That one-hour class became my sanctuary. They were evening classes, so there were no babies on the scene. I would see frantic new mums arrive to class, feeling stressed at leaving their partner to hold the fort or guilty for leaving their crying baby. They spent an hour in that class moving and looking after themselves, which is a rare opportunity in those early years. They left smiling, looking relaxed, looking more confident and hopefully holding a little less guilt. One thing to remind yourself is to not rush into it. Take it slow, go with how your body feels in each class – and find a good teacher!

fatigue, digestive issues, menstrual pain or irregularities, skin and hair problems are all signs of postnatal depletion. We put it to one side and then wonder why seven years later we're *still* not feeling quite like our 'old selves' yet. If you can imagine a bigger picture over the course of time – one, two, three pregnancies and births, breastfeeding, plus maybe fertility treatment or a couple of miscarriages along the way – you will start to see the impact of this continued hormone flux and depletion through a longer-term lens. Postnatal depletion can feel quite shocking, particularly if you were used to prioritising your fitness before you had children. Left unchecked, it can have profound mental health repercussions.

You need to be curious about why, if you're not feeling 'quite right', and stop saying, 'It'll be fine…'. Let's reject the 'bounce back' culture, but also let's not accept postnatal issues as being 'just the way it is when you've had a baby'.

Postnatal depression (PND)

PND symptoms clinically exist on a spectrum from mild towards extreme postpartum psychosis. If you feel you're experiencing what is, *for you,* unusual or unprecedented levels of guilt, self-doubt, anxiety, anger, fatigue, tearfulness, low mood and irritability, these are all worthy of investigation, without shame or embarrassment. PND may arrive 'out of the blue' when your baby is tiny, or might've been triggered by your birth experience (although *see* 'Birth trauma', p. 95, which is distinct and should be treated differently if you seek therapy for it). It can be heavily influenced by your temperament, and that of your baby – excessive crying has a detrimental impact on your mental health – as well as factors such as the amount of sleep you're getting, the support you have around you and your vulnerability to depression from past emotional experiences, such as your fertility journey or previous loss. A 2015 study quoted in the *Guardian* suggested that for some women PND symptoms peak *four years* after having a baby. It's not necessarily a black fog that envelops when you have a newborn, but instead may be more a cumulative effect of physical depletion and your emotional resilience being chipped away over time.

If you're feeling under par, just not like 'you', as if you're watching your life through mottled glass, be honest with yourself and reach out to someone close to you. It doesn't have to be your GP, just take the first step by voicing your feelings to someone. You may not have 'classic' depression symptoms, such as lack of bonding with your baby or withdrawing from the world, you may *look like* you're coping just fine. It may present for you as overwhelming anxiety, an incredibly loud inner critic, crippling self-doubt or excessive rage at your partner. Please seek help, there should be no stigma with reaching out for guidance in this time: I've provided useful sources of support in the Resources. You're not alone.

Protecting your mental and emotional health

Postnatal depression is still surrounded in stigma and taboo, but it shouldn't be. As symptoms appear on a spectrum from mild to severe, often we plough through, feeling like 'it's not as serious' as depression, so we don't admit to ourselves or others that we're struggling. The NCT have highlighted mental health issues in early motherhood with their 2017 Hidden Half campaign (*see* Resources for the web address). The report suggested that *half* the mums interviewed had mental or emotional problems, but were either too embarrassed or ashamed to admit this, or those who had approached their GP or health visitor had not received adequate support or information. This means that many women are left dealing with a mental health condition on their own, which, alongside the general hectic overwhelm of new motherhood, can present many issues of isolation and loneliness.

So, the first step is *noticing* how you're feeling. Taking note of your mental landscape is so vital, but as a mum you often slip so far down your list of priorities as to be usurped by the neighbour's dog. Depletion, if left unchecked, leaves you susceptible to depression.

How can Pilates help you experience a mentally healthy motherhood?

The psychological benefits of making time for movement and focusing on your wellbeing can't be underestimated. It's even more important now that your 'me time' has been downgraded to 'solo loo trip' as opposed to 'luxury spa weekend'. Pilates encourages you to take time, to press pause, to concentrate on how you're feeling, physically. Healing the body lends itself also to creating space for the mind – something that for mums can be in short supply.

Alongside Pilates, I teach mindfulness. Mindfulness-Based Cognitive Therapy (MBCT) is the NICE-recommended therapy for depression and anxiety, which is proven to enhance wellbeing and alleviate stress. Mindfulness is easily slotted into the mayhem of motherhood – you can be mindful at softplay or with your baby sitting on your head. There are a couple of meditations included within the book – have a play around with them, you never know, you might find this offers you the tiny moment of headspace that you've been craving.

My own postnatal experience

I have two brilliant, bonkers boys. First time around, I was a teeny bit smug going into motherhood. I taught Pilates. My career was in the strength of my abs. I had worked with pregnancy and postnatal clients for a few years, I thought I'd be guaranteed to recover quickly with all my amazing knowledge and practice – how could I not ping back into shape immediately, it was my job after all? I was certain I'd ease back into bodywork as a natural priority, when my baby slept through the night from about six weeks old… Yes. I had a complete fantasy in my head, and the reality was a big fat shock for body and mind.

My first birth was a traumatic affair: I went overdue by two weeks, developed pre-eclampsia, was induced and gave birth by crash Caesarean after a three-day labour. This all meant I embarked on my motherhood journey battered and exhausted, having had not a wink of sleep over a period of four days, and major abdominal surgery. My baby was also traumatised by his birth experience (he wasn't breathing when he came out) and severely underweight due to undiagnosed placental issues. Our first few months earthside together were characterised by a lot of crying and no sleep. This kind of birth experience is maybe on the extreme end but sadly not abnormal; indeed, it has been accepted as being quite common. Even the most natural, positive, 'perfect' of births can leave you feeling physically shaken, bruised and weak.

I was fully in survival mode for many months post birth. I didn't consciously breathe, I hardly ever drank any water, there was one particular newborn day when I ordered a pizza at 3p.m. as I hadn't eaten all day, with my crying baby in my arms.

My postnatal experience was like a forest fire in terms of a total loss of my fitness. When my son was two months old I tried to do a simple Knee Fold (*see* p. 71). I couldn't. I didn't have the strength in my abdominals to even lift one leg up off the floor without pain in my scar. I experienced lots of problems with my scar healing, and severe sleep deprivation for over a year meant that I simply couldn't face the idea of exercise. Sadly, I subsequently also had two miscarriages, and with the depletion resulting from that, I fairly inevitably developed postnatal depression. Stripped of all my strength – and forever my smugness – I had to build myself physically and emotionally back from nothing. This made me realise that no postnatal journey is simple or predictable. Yet mums are still under relentless pressure to 'bounce back' and 'get back to normal'.

My youngest is four. Second time round, I hit a different obstacle to my postnatal health and fitness. After a happily more positive birth experience and much easier initial recovery, I competed in a triathlon when he was six months old. It was great in lots of ways: it gave me a focus and ensured I prioritised exercise time – an escape from the mayhem of being a mum of two in those first intense six months. But it was too much too soon. My body simply wasn't ready. I injured my knee and then my shoulder. I hadn't rebuilt the fundamental strength in my inner core and glutes (bum) enough for the extra demands I was placing on them

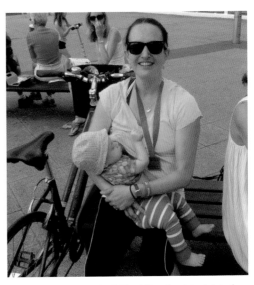

Anya giving 6-month old Freddie a feed straight after finishing the London Triathlon.

with training *and* motherhood. It then took over a year of rebuilding and rehabilitation to correct the damage I'd caused by being mega keen to 'get back to it'.

Looking back, I understand I needed to do a triathlon to prove I could do it, to be STRONG and avoid going through what had happened last time. But if I could do it over again, I would have focused on much more patient, careful, SLOW and steady core restoration. I should have seen a women's health physio for a complete body check before I even thought about high-impact exercise. This book is the culmination of seven years of my own postnatal rebuilding. I'm not 'done' – I'm still on that journey with you.

My experience, and the experiences of the many hundreds of postnatal clients I've had the privilege to work with over the past 10 years, is where the rehab exercises in this book come from. If you're a beginner with no background in Pilates or exercise, this is a perfect introduction for you. If you're a buggy runner eager to lose the mum tum and get back to 'normal' – whatever that may be – this is the ideal groundwork for you, too. Pilates is a fantastic tool in your postnatal healing and strength toolkit. The beauty of the method is that it is so applicable to help you in a functional way, to equip you for the physical and mental strength you need day to day.

Remember that even a supreme athlete like Serena Williams encountered struggles after birth. She lost her

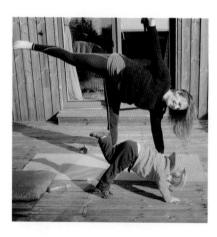

Anya and 2-year old Maurice doing some yoga play.

Wimbledon Final in 2018, 10 months after giving birth, saying, 'For all the moms out there, I was playing for you today. And I tried.' For a lot of us even the idea of picking up a tennis racquet, let alone possessing the stamina and springiness required for championship tennis, would have been a fantasy at 10 months postnatal. Motherhood is tough, and you're not alone if you're finding it challenging to build your strength.

Postnatal issues, if not addressed, become lifelong issues. *You are forever postnatal.* It's not a state you pass through for six weeks: it's what you are. We need to see our postnatal energy reboot as a long-term, ongoing project. Consider your body, fitness and wellbeing as a building-from-scratch project. It's all very well having grand plans for what wonderful interior decorating we want to do, but first, you need to build the four walls. This is brick by brick building the foundations for your long-term health and fitness. If you're not mindful of your body and fail to set aside time to heal, repair and recover, it's like forgetting to rebuild a supporting wall you've knocked down. Let's not paint before the plaster is dry. We need to rebuild on multiple levels, and some days/weeks/months may feel harder than others. This book will provide you with the information you need to build the strongest foundations (and, happily, the peachiest bum).

Your long-term postnatal healing

There are certain things that you will have to soften into accepting once you're a mum. These are:

- *Scars*, changes to sensation or long-term effects from birth injuries/ nerve damage – Some birth experiences bring with them scars we can't simply delete, and scar tissue may create issues with sensation in the long term. But we can soften and accept, connect to our bodies, do our best to listen and be kind to it. *You're allowed to love your body.* Try not to waste energy being hateful of your body. Model self-love for your children – how would you feel if they viewed themselves through constantly critical eyes? Are they mirroring something that they see all the time from your attitude to yourself? Consider how powerful it would be if we dwelled on things we loved about ourselves rather than what we hated.

- *Stretch marks* – Mexican midwives call these 'love lines' – wouldn't it be kinder if we saw them as 'love lines' rather than ugly marks on our body?

- *Changes to your boobs* – Breastfeeding and hormonal changes of pregnancy can wreak havoc on your assets and this is something that we may have to accept as a part of our body's shifting into motherhood. Posture is everything: standing tall can make even the droopiest boobs look more pert. And a good supportive (comfortable) bra works wonders.

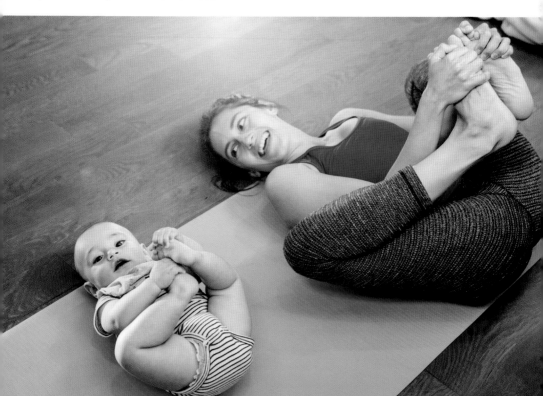

- *Heightened emotion and anxiety* – These are part of the physiological changes that we undergo, enabling us to be the mama cat, always ready to protect our young. Breathing helps to soothe your nervous system into understanding when anxiety is creating fictional stories for you, but be reassured that you are not being 'neurotic', 'hormonal' or overemotional, you are being a mum, and heightened emotions are your mum power.

There are, however, some things that you absolutely should NOT accept as 'just part of being a mum':

- *Diastasis recti* (abdominal separation, *see* p. 44) and long-term weakness in your core. My first midwife, palpating my 26-week bump said darkly 'you have very strong abdominals – they won't ever be that way again after you've had your baby!' I was a bit upset by her negativity – people don't see the power of a flippant comment when you're pregnant and vulnerable. As long as you know you have diastasis recti and work towards healing it correctly, you can absolutely regain your strength.

- *Incontinence and pelvic organ prolapse.* Peeing your pants even a little bit when you jump, run, sneeze, cough? A feeling of heaviness in your vagina as if you're 'falling out'? Just part of being a mum? Nope. *Absolutely not.* And you shouldn't ignore it or grab a pad and put up with it. As a culture we have somehow normalised postnatal incontinence, we laugh it off as if it's hilarious. But this does our longer-term physical and mental health no favours at all. Pelvic floor dysfunction may be common straight after you've had a baby, *but it is not normal* in the long term, and shouldn't be accepted … remember you have so much of your life still ahead of you. Honour your 75-year old self by doing something about this issue today. In the UK, the government have just announced that as part of their 10-year plan for the NHS women will see a physiotherapist as standard after having a baby, following the practice of countries such as France. But until this is fully implemented, you will have to take more responsibility for your own recovery – and this book will help you to do that.

- *Fatigue.* Fatigue is a heavy coat we wear while bringing our little ones up. In the early years of sleep deprivation and the relentless rush hour of small children, it is arguably inevitable. Show me a new mum without dark eye circles and I would surmise an Instagram filter was at play. Try to implement self-care strategies to ensure fatigue doesn't become a permanent houseguest. Rest (even closing your eyes for 10 full seconds can count as rest in the early days). Breathing. Meditation. Adequate hydration, good nutrition, movement and fresh air, green space. Checking your

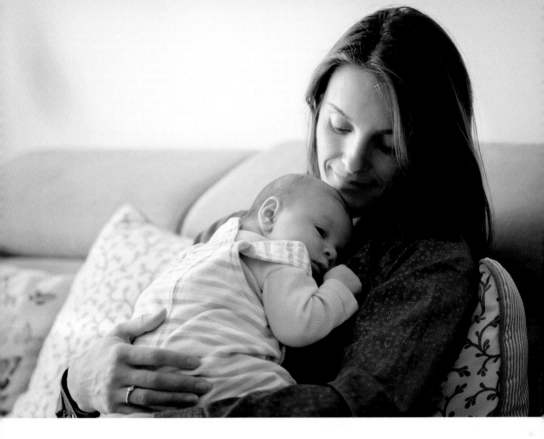

mineral levels such as iron and zinc to ensure your organs and digestion are firing properly. Fatigue is something motherhood brings with it in spades – even once they start sleeping through the night gloriously, there'll be a regression of some sort somewhere down the line. Your postnatal healing journey isn't a linear one step forwards two steps back, but more one step forwards, two steps sideways, a leap back … etc. The unpredictability of the early years of motherhood definitely takes its toll on your energy levels. But fatigue isn't something you should put up with long term without question. It's worth bearing in mind that fatigue is a core symptom of depression. So it may be that your lethargy and tiredness is your body trying to communicate something to you that needs addressing. Your body speaks your mind.

This book will help you build your strength for the long term, step by step, in three stages:

- **Stage 1: Awareness –** *Mind–muscle connection.* You can't strengthen what you can't feel or connect to. In the early weeks and months you may have a desire to 'get back into it'. But you'll reap the biggest rewards if you properly work on your muscle awareness first. Releasing tension allows you to *connect* properly, and only then will the real strength follow.

- **Stage 2: Foundations** – Once you can activate that deep connection with your core, *we have to practise and challenge it in movement.* **Stage 2** exercises focus on maintaining stability with varying degrees of challenge of load and coordination. This helps you to train for *life*: to find that activation in *functional situations* – while picking up your baby or putting your toddler in the car seat, for example. It's crucial to spend enough time here at **Stage 2** before you take on high-impact exercise.

- **Stage 3: Build on it** – Once you've found, then activated your core, then you can begin to challenge yourself more to grow *stronger*. Often, mums feel like they plateau with their recovery and don't seem to feel/see that elusive core strength or tummy tone. Maybe you're staying at a comfort zone at Stage 2 and not offering yourself *enough* demand on your muscles. But if you're still leaking while you run, it means you've headed straight for **Stage 3** without spending enough quality time at Stages 1 and 2. Don't be scared to challenge yourself *when the time is right.* Muscle needs progressive challenge to build itself up and be stronger. Progress, just do it consciously and with patience – listen to your body, notice responses to different loads of challenge (e.g., if that made me leak wee/my tummy gap dome, it's too soon to try that), and adapt accordingly.

Miss any of the steps, skip the foundations, and you'll end up looping back round to the beginning at some point through injury or pelvic floor dysfunction. Similarly, if you stay comfortably at Stage 2, you might feel frustrated after a long time and wonder why you're not feeling stronger.

Let's get started!

Tip

You'll find **Stages 1** and **2** in chapters 1–3, and **Stage 3** in chapters 4–5. Taking the time to carefully notice and adjust your daily breathing, and postural and movement patterns will be much more beneficial in the long run to your core strength and ability to 'lose your baby weight' than jumping enthusiastically into a Buggy Runners group straight after your 'six-week sign off', when your insides may be like soft blancmange.

Chapter 1

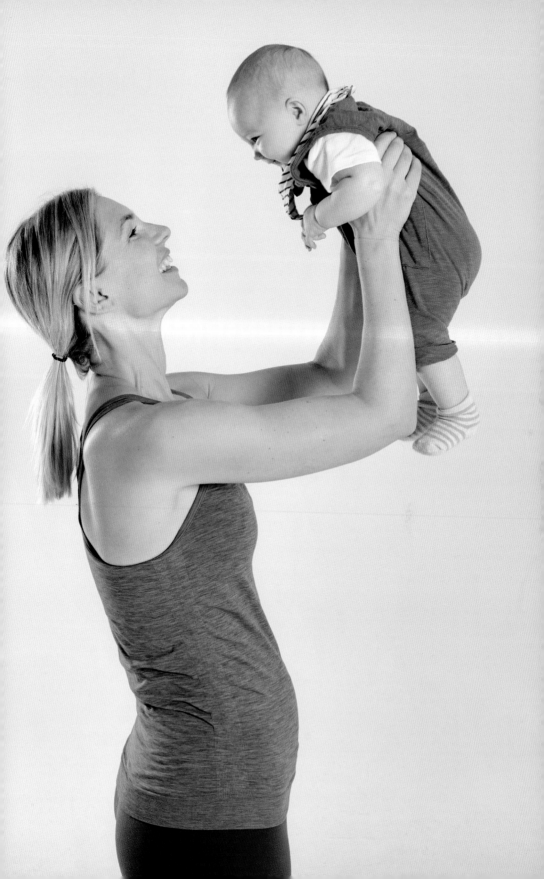

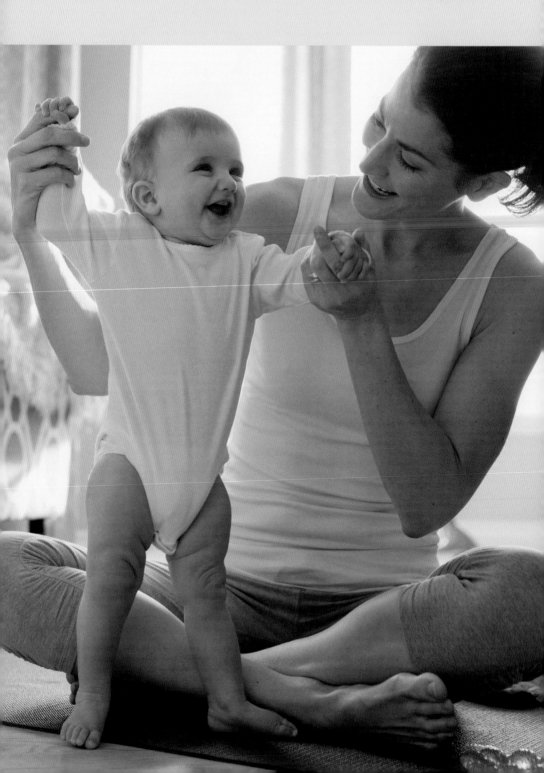

Pilates fundamentals

How pregnancy, birth and motherhood challenge the body

Welcome to Motherland! After having a baby, society seems preoccupied with getting you back into your pre-pregnancy jeans *looking* fantastic, rather than back home into your body *feeling* well and functioning normally again. As long as you've 'bounced back', society doesn't seem to mind if you're weeing yourself when you sneeze. This chapter gives you an overview of the changes that birth and motherhood bring to your body and introduces the basic fundamentals of Pilates to show how this amazing body-conditioning programme can help rebuild our strength and counterbalance the effects of birth on the body. The exercises in this chapter form your foundation of Pilates and are appropriate for all postnatal stages. The following chapters then present a progressive Pilates programme for specific needs of each postnatal stage of recovery over the first year (and beyond).

The 'bounce back' culture is disrespectful to the vast changes that have happened within your body, emotions and brain over the course of pregnancy and from your childbirth experience. Moving into motherhood is a whole-body and mind transformation: a *matrescence*. This is a term that was coined in the 1970s by the anthropologist Dana Raphael to describe the period of transition – in mind, body and spirit – that women enter when they have a baby. Birthing a baby also births the mother. It's akin to adolescence in the scale of hormonal intensity and body changes, and yet culturally we don't view it with the same understanding of it being a huge metamorphosis. Look at reproductive psychiatrist Dr Alexandra Sacks' wonderful TED talk on this time of change (details in the Resources). Just as adolescence brings with it an earthquake of physical and emotional changes, so does *matrescence*.

Motherhood presents a time where there is more change to brain activity than at any other stage in a woman's life. Our brain shrinks slightly in later pregnancy, and these changes are thought to last for around two years after pregnancy. Our brains literally become restructured, fine-tuned to the skills needed once the baby is born. Emotional intelligence areas grow to ensure we can be empathetic and respond to our baby's needs. Your amygdala, the 'lizard', ancient brain, is one of the greatest beneficiaries of these changes, but this also means that your fight-or-flight (anxiety) response is heightened.

It makes perfect sense: you are now the protector of your young, but it can be an unexpected – and uncomfortable – change, particularly if you've never particularly experienced anxiety before. Consider it a brain upgrade, new software to deal with the greater demands being placed on it.

For a detailed outline of the brain and other physiological changes, see Dr Oscar Serrallach's 2018 book *The Postnatal Depletion Cure*. The changes that we experience are profound and potentially long lasting. These are perfectly legitimate reasons to feel a bit low or weak, and yet we don't prioritise our healing recovery. Kimberly Ann Johnson, author of the wonderful book *The Fourth Trimester*, likens modern postnatal recovery to the mentality we have if we fall over in the street: we get up immediately, eyes down, and speed off quickly to avoid embarrassment or attention, and like a cat, lick our wounds alone in private. Actually, we need to sit and breathe for a moment to assess the damage – or even better, be vulnerable and reach for help to get back up.

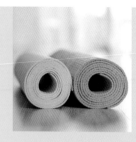

CASE STUDY

Julie, mum of three

I was really cynical about Pilates initially as I've previously enjoyed high-impact workouts and running as my exercise. I felt that if I didn't have trouble breathing and wasn't dripping in sweat, then how could I really be exercising! But I found that very quickly my back pain eased.

I felt my core strengthening and noticed improvements in my breathing when I did other forms of exercise. The results were noticeable almost immediately. Also, I felt challenged, but at an attainable level.

What's going on in my body?

Here's a timeline of what to expect in the first year post birth, from the early days.

DAYS 1 TO 10

What to expect:

- Night sweats – loss of extra fluids, particularly if you had lots of swelling in late pregnancy. Expect to soak through your nightclothes in bodily fluids.
- Heavy bleeding.
- Discomfort/pain from pelvic floor trauma or Caesarean scar.
- Your blood pressure, heart rate, body temperature and breathing gradually return to normal over this time.
- Your boobs will go through huge changes as your milk comes in, whether you breastfeed or not. They may grow to an alarming size and become painfully rock hard. This will pass, but make sure you massage your boobs if you feel they are uncomfortably hard and full, and put baby on your breast as often as you can (even overnight) to establish breastfeeding and relieve the milk build-up to regulate your supply.
- Your nipples may be very sore and tender. This is normal even if breastfeeding is going well. Breathe deeply and slowly while feeding. The pain will settle soon. Be aware of the symptoms of thrush and mastitis (I've provided a link to the relevant NHS webpage in the Resources), and seek medical attention as soon as you can if necessary.
- Mood swings, heightened anxiety: often called the 'baby blues'. There is a huge hormonal watershed now that you no longer have the placenta creating hormones for you, and you begin to return to pre-pregnancy hormone levels within the body. You may feel euphoric one moment and tearful the next. You may feel elated, or defeated by your birth experience. You may feel chaotic due to hormonal fluctuation and emotional intensity/sleep deprivation. All of these feelings are common and normal, but worth tracking in case they linger for longer than a short period of time.
- Urinary incontinence, especially when sneezing or coughing.
- If you had a C-section, flatulence and painful trapped wind are to be expected.

Safe exercises for this stage:

- Pelvic floor awareness exercises.
- Breathing: deep, long, full breaths.
- Ankle circles, pointing and flexing your feet, foot exercises (*see* p. 51), Legs Up the Wall (*see* p. 114), neck and shoulder stretches: gentle, restorative, soothing movement.
- If you had a C-section: gentle coughs to stimulate the area around the stitches.

DAYS 10 TO 21

What to expect:

- Lighter bleeding.
- Healing around C-section and episiotomy should be progressing well but may still be painful, swollen and bruised.
- If C-section, the scar site will probably be numb and tender. It will hurt to cough, sneeze, laugh. Remember to take your pain medication.
- Your nipples will probably still be very sore if you are breastfeeding. Keep nipple cream in the fridge and apply liberally in between feeds. Allow your nipples to 'air dry' where possible. Breastmilk has magic powers for healing so squeeze some on your own nipples if they are really sore.
- Pregnant tummy will still be prominent.
- Healing still going on at deep level: organs are reassembling within your abdomen.

Safe exercises for this stage:

- Stay low intensity. When lifting your baby/carrying toddlers and when getting up off the floor, consciously *breathe out and lift up your pelvic floor* to support your effort.
- Avoid strenuous aerobic exercise for the first six weeks, even if you feel raring to go. Walking is fine.
- Your pelvic floor may still be sore and you may still be leaking when you sneeze/cough. Practise finding the pelvic floor muscles on an exhalation: and try to remember to lift your pelvic floor just before you cough or sneeze.

WEEKS FOUR TO SIX

What to expect:

- There may still be some wound healing/scar pain and discomfort.
- Pain from establishing breastfeeding should have settled by now – if it hasn't, seek some advice and help about checking your baby's latch. Details in the Resources.
- Bleeding should have completely stopped by now.
- By the end of this period your uterus has contracted back to its pre-pregnancy size, which can feel very painful; it is often more painful and happens more quickly with second and subsequent births.
- Your tummy may still look quite pregnant due to the stretching of your abdominal muscles and skin.

Safe exercises for this stage:

- Gentle, low-impact movement, Pilates, stretching, yoga – but be cautious of intense held stretches and avoid hot yoga, as ligaments will still be vulnerable due to pregnancy hormone levels still levelling off: the hormone relaxin increases the laxity of your joints.
- Moderate-intensity low-impact exercise: longer walks, cycling.

WEEKS SIX TO EIGHT

What to expect:

- Sleep deprivation accumulation may affect energy levels.
- Back, neck and shoulder aches and wrist pains are common due to repetitive movements in early motherhood.
- Hair may begin to fall out due to hormonal levels returning to pre-pregnancy levels (dependent on breastfeeding – if you're breastfeeding your hormones may take a bit longer to recalibrate to pre-pregnancy levels).
- Pelvic pain may still be present if experienced during pregnancy, particularly if breastfeeding. Beware of starting HIIT or running in an effort to 'bounce back' at this stage as pelvic floor weakness will still be present and pelvic joints are vulnerable to injury.
- You may have your GP check – ask to be referred to a women's health physio for a full physical check. *All* women should ideally be seen by a physio postnatally. This model of postnatal care is in the workings for the standard pathway of care in the next 10 years, but isn't standard as yet so you'll need to ask.

Safe exercises for this stage:

- Pelvic floor and stability exercises, Pelvic Tilts (*see* p. 57).
- Lots of stretching and opening shoulders. Lying on the floor, palms facing up, can be very beneficial.
- Low-impact cardio: walking, gentle cycling, swimming – although avoid breaststroke if experiencing pelvic pain or discomfort.
- Build in enough rest, deep breathing and stretching to release tension.
- Begin gentle abdominal massage (*see* p. 124).

MONTHS TWO TO THREE

What to expect:

- Chronic tiredness and fatigue may begin to affect your mental health and resilience.
- If you're chronically tired and have low energy even though your baby has started sleeping a bit more then it may not purely be due to sleep deprivation, so go to your GP and request an iron and other mineral levels check. Now's a good time to check in with your diet, if you haven't already. Are you optimising your nutrient intake?
- If you have access to one, now is the ideal time to go to a women's health physio to have a whole-body check: pelvic floor, abdominals, breathing, posture.
- Diastasis recti (DR): the greatest time of natural healing of abdominal separation occurs in the first eight weeks. After eight weeks the process of automatic healing slows down. *See* p. 44 for more about DR.

Safe exercises for this stage:

- Pelvic floor, pelvic floor, pelvic floor.
- Have your diastasis recti checked by a professional — and begin targeted deep abdominal recovery exercises.
- Avoid planks and sit-ups in favour of gentle but targeted core restore Pilates — standing, bending, squatting, side lying, all fours.
- Avoid running until cleared by a women's health physio. Do NOT run at all yet if you are leaking urine. It doesn't mean never again, it just means not now.
- The postnatal GP check is not, and never has been, a 'clearance for exercise'. There is growing awareness of the fact that *all* women need to be seen for a physical check-up by a women's health physio, but particularly if they desire to get back into high-impact exercise such as HIIT or running. For the latest (2018) physio-led guidelines about returning to high-impact exercise postnatally, see the publication listed in the Resources. Pelvic organ prolapse risk is high at this stage (*see* p. 42).
- Stretch and release tension in neck, shoulders.

FOUR TO SIX MONTHS

What to expect:

- Tendency to gain weight, particularly if breastfeeding/energy levels are very low, or if still suffering from incontinence and scared to exercise.
- You should hopefully be feeling physically a bit 'more normal'.
- Aches and pains are common: neck, back, shoulder, hips, due to the repetitive movements of motherhood and lack of stretching.
- Your periods may have returned by now, even if you're exclusively breastfeeding (unfair, right?). It's important to be aware that you can still get pregnant while breastfeeding, so if returning to sexual activity you need to consider contraception.
- Your uterus stretches during pregnancy, so it's common for periods to be much heavier after pregnancy due to the extra surface area of the uterus. See your GP if you're concerned about particularly heavy bleeding.

Safe exercises for this stage:

- Pelvic floor — *important even if you had a C-section*.
- Aerobic exercise. Bear in mind the fragile energy-balance equation: tiredness can be counterbalanced with exercise, and sleep/anxiety symptoms may be improved by exercise. But if you are exhausted and depleted, proper rest is more beneficial (meditation/reading/breathing and stretching, instead of scrolling on your phone when baby naps, etc).
- If you are still experiencing urinary incontinence, please don't delay seeing a physio. Ask to be referred by your GP. Weeing yourself is common but not normal. *Do not do high-impact exercise while still leaking: it won't get better if you 'push through' it.*

- Be mindful of potential ligament laxity and avoid wide-legged unstable HIIT moves such as Skaters if they feel uncomfortable in the pelvis.
- Focus on glute strengthening alongside pelvic floor/deep abdominal activation work.

SIX MONTHS TO ONE YEAR

What to expect:

- You may feel your mojo returning, depending on how much sleep you're getting. It may take longer – everyone is on a different healing journey so don't compare.
- Keep an eye on your mental health. Depression and anxiety can begin to take hold once the intensity of the newborn phase is over and as a result of the cumulative effects of sleep deprivation. Don't be scared to reach out for support.
- Focus on your posture, breathing and how you *feel inside* rather than on weight loss or gain.
- It is also normal NOT to feel as strong as you were pre baby yet. Aches and pains from baby duties are common, your baby is getting heavier by the day and more challenging. You are still very newly postnatal in the grand scheme of things.

Safe exercises for this stage:

- Walking, swimming and low-impact cardio are very valuable for your physical and mental health.
- Returning to your pre-pregnancy levels of activity is safe so long as there are no pelvic floor and diastasis recti issues. However...
- You're more vulnerable to injury right now, so literally don't run before you can walk.
- Stretching, conscious resting, such as meditation, and deep breathing cannot be underestimated in value.

ONE YEAR TO FOREVER

- *You are still postnatal.*
- Be gentle with yourself. If you're frustrated with 'how far you've come', remember postnatal strength and recovery is often not linear. It's common to experience setbacks.

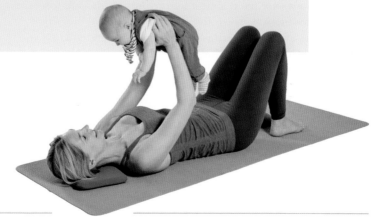

Your birthing body – what happens in your body during birth?

Your pelvis

The pelvis is a pretty amazing design. It's made up of four bones, arranged like a fused bony ring at the bottom of your spine. You can locate certain parts of your pelvis by palpating your skin: at the front you can find the **ilium bone**; the **iliac crest** is the bony parts of your hips; at the front is your **anterior-superior iliac spine** (or ASIS); and at the back, your **posterior-superior iliac spine** (PSIS).

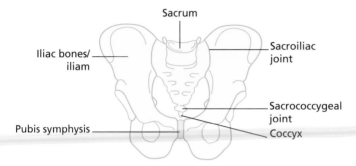

Your **ischia** are your sit bones – the oft forgotten bones that we tend to curl underneath us rather than actually sitting on. At the back, you can feel the triangular-shaped bony pattern of the **sacrum**, which ends in the **coccyx**, the remains of our tail. In the front is the **pubic bone**, which is in fact two bones, one from the left side of the pelvis and one from the right, fused together by thick fibrous cartilage.

Take some time to orientate yourself with your own pelvis. Get a sense of the width of your pelvis, the height, its relation to your ribcage. The pelvis is the seat of your power, and postnatally is the key to unlocking a lot of imbalances that flow through the body.

What happens to the pelvic bones during birth?

When not affected by hormones, the pelvic ligaments connecting the pelvic bones are fixed almost like grouting, allowing for minimal movement between the joints. Like the engineering of a bridge, some movement is necessary to react adequately to pressures of temperature, wind and load, but too much would compromise the strength of the bridge. Pregnancy hormonal changes ensure that these ligaments become more lax, which means the bones have a movement potential previously not allowed. If you suffered from pelvic girdle pain (PGP) you may be painfully aware of this.

The laxity is one of the miracles of the human body: during a vaginal birth this is how your baby is able to wriggle their way out of the birth canal. The pubic symphysis makes very small sliding and opening movements. The sacroiliac joints allow for a greater opening for the head to enter into the pelvis. The base of the sacrum moves backwards and the coccyx forwards. The iliac crests (hip bones) spread, which opens the top of the pelvis. Then, as your baby descends, the sit bones open, which triggers all of the preceding movements to reverse, like doors closing after baby exits. Imagine a time-lapse video of a flower opening and expanding, then closing – this is exactly what happens to your amazing, brilliant pelvis to allow your baby into the world. No wonder you may feel like you've been hit by a bus afterwards.

Your pelvic floor

The pelvic floor isn't just one muscle. It's a group of muscles: interlinked, overlapping and webbed together in a figure-of-eight shape around your anus, vagina and urethra, ensuring your bladder, uterus and bowel have a strict turnstile to get through before they can empty. The pelvic floor works in delicate balance with your abdominals, diaphragm, back muscles and glute (buttock) muscles that stabilise the pelvis – in other words, your pelvic floor influences and is influenced by *the whole of your body*. Men also have a pelvic floor, but they have only two orifices (the anus and urethra), and no baby exit route to consider – and therefore they don't tend to suffer the pelvic floor trauma early on in their lives that women do.

Our pelvic floors go through a lot. Nine months (maybe slightly more) of pregnancy strains the muscles' resilience. Any sickness you experienced places great additional pressure on the muscles, so if you suffered severe sickness throughout your pregnancy, such as hyperemesis gravidarum (HG), you may well have weakened your pelvic floor significantly before you had your baby.

Your pelvic floor, diaphragm and abdominal muscles together use huge strength during contractions to push your baby down through the pelvic cavity. The pressure your baby presents on the pelvic floor brings about a reflex contraction of the uterus,

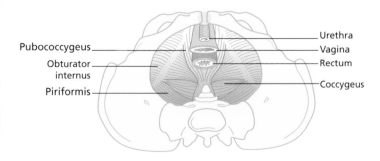

Pubococcygeus

Obturator internus

Piriformis

Urethra

Vagina

Rectum

Coccygeus

The pelvic floor muscles (female).

the expulsive reflex. This pressure, alongside these expulsive contractions cause the perineum to stretch, at first at the back because the head places most pressure at the coccyx to push out, and then at the front. Even for a Caesarean birth without labouring first, your pelvic floor has been your baby's trampoline for nine months.

In an ideal world, every new mum would see a women's health physio as a matter of course in a normal postnatal pathway of care, to make sure we're firing on all cylinders before we take on the world again post birth. This isn't *yet* part of our standard postnatal care, so we have to make sure we take responsibility for our own healing. The main thing to remember about your pelvic floor after birth is that you shouldn't suffer in silence. Pelvic floor issues simply do not get better if they are ignored. If you are struggling with pain, discomfort, lack of sensation, a feeling of 'bearing down'/'falling out', or simply if things don't feel 'normal' – *not* asking for help means that the problem will only get worse over time.

One of the most common pelvic floor issues is incontinence. The 2019 National Institute for Health and Care Excellence (NICE) guidelines for treating stress urinary incontinence, and pelvic floor dysfunction such as pelvic organ prolapse (*see* p. 42) advise that women should be offered 'a trial of supervised pelvic floor muscle training of at least 3 months' duration as first-line treatment'. In a trial study conducted in 2018 by BMC *Women's Health,* women suffering from incontinence were offered pelvic physiotherapy alongside tailored Pilates classes for 12 weeks, and the results showed, 'a range of benefits for women who attended Pilates classes … had lower symptom severity … improved self-esteem, decreased social embarrassment and lower impact on normal daily activities… Women with higher symptom severity showed improvement in their personal relationships.' The data also indicated that Pilates classes, 'could positively influence attitudes to exercise, diet and wellbeing.' So you're absolutely in the right place here.

Pelvic floor exercises

So Pilates can help with your pelvic floor. What does that actually *mean?* You've probably been told you need to 'strengthen your pelvic floor'. You might have been squeezing hopefully, eyebrows raised, clenching everything – your bum, your thighs, your jaw? To retrain your pelvic floor for life after birth, pelvic floor *awareness* – learning to isolate only your pelvic floor and not grip the muscles that surround it, and knowing how to fully release as well as squeeze – is vital. And this awareness takes time to tune into.

Your pelvic floor strength is affected by how you move and carry yourself (and carry your children) every day. *Movement* stimulates your pelvic floor – so in this respect, every exercise in this book, and everything you do every day, is a pelvic floor exercise: stretching, toning, stimulating the floor through movement and breathing. That's also why sitting a lot isn't great for the pelvic floor: it deprives it of movement and circulation; a sedentary lifestyle isn't good news for pelvic floor health.

Pelvic floor 'exercises' – where you rhythmically lift and release your pelvic floor muscles – are really important for postnatal healing and are profoundly effective, *when done correctly*. But we tend to think they're boring, aren't quite sure if we're doing it right and so we skip them, which makes us feel guilty. Guilt and boredom – not really a magical combination, right? But actually, these exercises are the secret seasoning in the recipe for a vibrant life. You need them now more than you've ever needed them. Don't see them as boring. Or, if they *are* boring for you, it's the same boring that brushing your teeth is – something that you wouldn't dream of forgoing or not making time for. They are part of essential life upkeep. Imagine if from now on you didn't brush your teeth every day, twice a day. What would your teeth look and feel like, aged 75? Exactly the same principle applies to your pelvic floor health. Since you always remember to do one, why not try doing the other at the same time?

The way the human body was designed means that we shouldn't need to 'exercise' our pelvic floor – we should be utilising its strength naturally through daily effort and movement. However, modern humans have a very convenient comfortable captive life where we now really don't need to move that much (hello, sitting

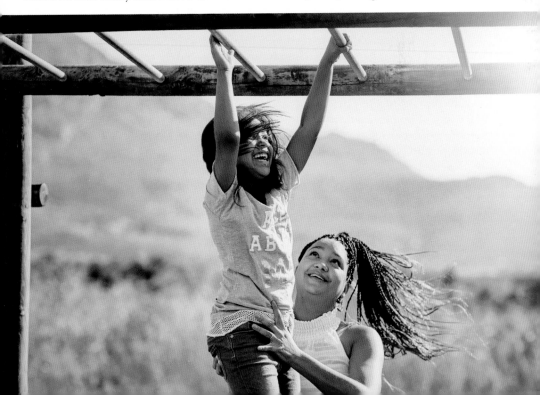

at a desk for 8 hours) or go that far under our own steam. We use a tiny fraction of the physical strength that our prehistoric ancestors needed on a daily basis to survive. We don't climb, swing, jump, run or walk the way our bodies were meant to (and, indeed, the way children's playgrounds encourage our children to). Once we're adults, we generally sit on our bums quite a lot and eat biscuits.

Yet all movement, all of the power we need for the lifting, pushing, pulling etc in our daily lives stems from healthy pelvic floor function and its related synchronicities within the body. What's more, the pelvic floor is the last line of defence to ensure our organs (and fluids) are safely held inside. So you can see that when you add the hormonal and physical demands of childbirth and motherhood that without a fully effective pelvic floor this defence will be poor. Luckily, becoming more aware of your breathing and of your alignment will quite quickly have a positive effect on your natural pelvic floor function, improve your daily movement patterns and lessen the general strain on your joints.

Pelvic organ prolapse (POP)

There is a real risk of pelvic organ prolapse postnatally. A prolapse is when the uterus, bowel or bladder descends into the vagina. Some studies have found that 50 per cent of women will suffer from a prolapse post birth (Hagen et al 2004) – and often it happens in the three-month period when people are keen to jump back into exercising to lose baby weight. It is so important to strengthen your pelvic floor to help you avoid this. If you feel any sensation of your insides 'falling out', *do not ignore this.* Go to your GP and ask to be referred to a women's health physio. Pelvic organ prolapse can't always be prevented, but it can be managed.

Pelvic floor health declines as we age, particularly if we do nothing to maintain awareness and strength – this is one of those inevitable facts of life, like death and taxes. Staggeringly, only 25 per cent of women aged 18–83 have 'normal' pelvic floor support (Swift et al 2003). Much of this is arguably to do with lifestyle, postural habits and suffering in silence. So make sure you proactively do all you can to ensure that you strengthen your pelvic floor post birth, particularly if you know you want to have more children. It's not acceptable to be told that you should wait until you have completed your family before you can get proper help or be referred for surgery to 'fix' the problem. Statistics show that surgery without physiotherapy to help find the root cause of issues is rarely 100 per cent successful, with a significant chance of prolapse reoccurring. You need to strengthen as much as you can *between babies* otherwise you simply build more load on to an increasingly weaker foundation.

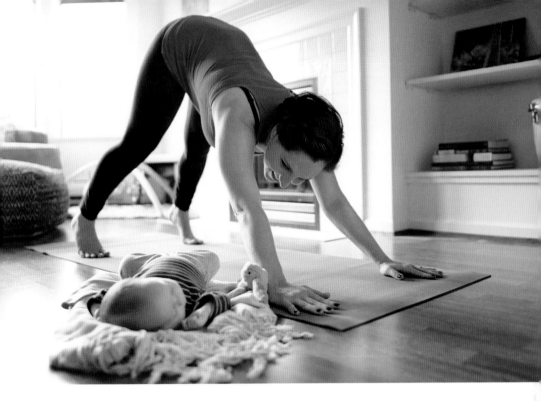

Pelvic floor dysfunction

Pelvic floor dysfunction makes itself apparent in a few ways. You may have lack of bladder control or lack of bowel control. You might wee a bit when you cough, sneeze laugh or run. You may have a desperate sudden need to run to the loo as soon as you turn your key in your lock when you get home. You may suffer from involuntarily breaking wind, which can feel excruciatingly embarrassing. Or constipation – and then straining on the loo causes even more pelvic floor and emotional issues. You may have pain, or a feeling of 'bearing down' during exercise or sex. All of these are symptoms of pelvic floor dysfunction. We shouldn't laugh it off. It shouldn't be something you're just expected to put up with after having a baby. We deserve better ladies. Pelvic floor health is not something we should accept will inevitably decline after having babies.

Hypertonicity

Hypertonicity is something that isn't widely understood as we're generally so obsessed with 'strengthening the pelvic floor'. When pelvic floor exercises are usually discussed, we only hear about 'squeezing', 'strengthening' and Kegels. But this misses out the full spectrum of recruitment for your pelvic floor muscles and can cause over-tightness. Consider your bicep muscles – they bend your arm in, but they can also *release* to straighten your arm out. You'd be a bit stuck if you could only hold your arm in a slightly bent 'strong' position, with neither of the two ends of the movement spectrum available to you. Sometimes strength is only half the story. We need softness, release, too: flexibility. This *flexible strength* is what we need in our pelvic floor.

Hypertonicity means excessive tone, tension or activity in the muscles – in other words, muscles held permanently in a 'tight' clenched position. Imagine walking around with a clenched fist all day. After a while, those muscles won't function as efficiently, and they'll fatigue and work incorrectly, causing you aches and pains. If this over-recruitment tightness happens to your pelvic floor, the muscles won't be able to function well.

Possible signs and symptoms of hypertonicity are: pain during sex; general soreness in the pelvic floor; pelvic pain; downward pressure in the vagina; pain when sitting; tightness, throbbing, aching, stabbing, spasm; bladder frequency; difficulty emptying the bladder and bowels; constipation. If you recognise any of these symptoms, visit a specialist pelvic health physiotherapist so you can start to remedy the situation.

In order to avoid hypertonicity, then, we need to learn to fully *release* the pelvic floor, as well as strengthen it. This is where breathing patterns are essential, as by breathing properly you learn to train the pelvic floor to release down as you inhale and to lift and work correctly with the abdominals as you exhale.

Pelvic floor restoration

To heal the pelvic floor we need to:

- **Realign:** Notice your posture, patterns of movement, incorrect muscle recruitment and correct them.
- **Release:** Let got of any tension you're holding on to in your pelvic area: abdominals/hips/glutes/pelvic floor.
- **Awareness:** Build your awareness of your pelvic floor and **connect** to it every day.
- **Strengthen:** Only after you have found your **connection**.

Remember: **Stage 1** = Awareness
           Stage 2 = Foundations
           Stage 3 = Build on it

Your abdominals: diastasis recti

Around the second trimester, depending on the size of your bump, you will have experienced some degree of abdominal separation: diastasis recti. The rectus abdominis muscle is your 'six-pack' muscle. It runs down your front, from your breastbone to your pubic bone: two segments running vertically parallel and intersected by a fibrous band, the linea alba.

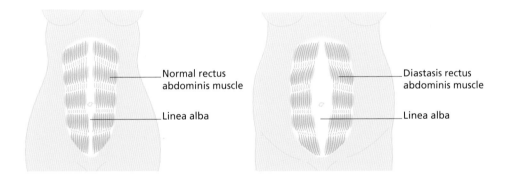

Normal rectus abdominis muscle

Linea alba

Diastasis rectus abdominis muscle

Linea alba

In a brilliant design feature that showcases the human body's adaptability, as your bump grew, the linea alba stretched to allow your baby more space; the two bands of muscle stretched away from the centre. Normally, the linea alba has a non-stretchy consistency without much 'give', almost like cotton. During pregnancy, however, hormonal activity ensures that it becomes more like Lycra, and responds to your bump's demand that it relaxes and stretches.

This is a normal structural adaptation, and you can't necessarily prevent it, and neither would you want to – it is a design feature specially created for your baby's comfort and growing power. Around 30 per cent of women experience this abdominal separation in the second trimester, with a further 66 per cent separating in the third trimester. Some research says that 100 per cent of women have some level of diastasis of the rectus abdominis by the third trimester (Gilliard and Brown 1996, Diane Lee 2013). Look at those stats again: *100 per cent of women have this happen at some point to some degree during pregnancy.*

The extent of your abdominal separation depends on a number of factors:

- your abdominal tone pre-pregnancy
- whether or not you carried more than one baby
- whether or not you've previously had more than one baby
- whether or not you put on a lot of weight, or carried a big baby – the latter will have had less space and needed to 'pop further out'
- your age: it can be worse if you're over 35
- your exercise and fitness levels
- the quality of your diet
- daily posture – are you stooping/lifting constantly without care for your technique and form?

Mind the gap

Until quite recently healthcare and fitness professionals have talked in terms of 'closing the gap'. But we now know that it's not the presence or even the *width* of the gap that's the issue:

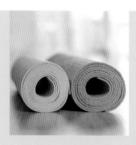

CASE STUDY

Miranda, mum of two

My diastasis recti gap wasn't very big each time and seemed to close pretty naturally but it was good to be aware of exercises I shouldn't do. The temptation with a wobbly tummy is to go straight into all the sit-up-type exercises to try to flatten the tummy, but these would have made it worse.

it's whether or not there is deep tone of the supporting muscles and fascia (connective tissue). So you could have a three-finger gap, but as long as your core muscles are firing properly and you can manage your intra-abdominal pressure – the pressure in the space between your respiratory system (your diaphragm) and your reproductive system, placing load out into your belly or down into your pelvic floor – this gap is considered to be 'functional', i.e. not a problem. You may *never* 'close the gap' completely, but as long as you have tone, this is OK.

A *problematic* diastasis recti is one where there's soft squishy tissue rather than tensile active tissue in the linea alba, therefore not supporting your core in movement, leaving you vulnerable to injury and pelvic floor issues. *See* p. 49 for the 'rec check', and for more detail about this.

Diastasis recti used to be considered a purely cosmetic issue – the 'mum tum' 'postnatal pooch' – and generally dismissed by GPs, 'well you've had a baby what do you expect? Do some sit-ups.' This has been very unhelpful for women. There is a direct correlation between a diastasis recti and the load placed on your pelvic floor and your spine. If you have a serious gap, this has an impact on the ability of your abdominals to control the balance of your pelvis and spine, with the result that you may also experience back pain and/or symptoms of pelvic floor dysfunction. (And you *shouldn't be doing sit-ups* as you'll make it worse.)

You might have noticed when you were pregnant that when you got out of bed or even up from sitting, there was a strange doming in your stomach, a bit like an alien pushing out, or a Toblerone-shaped triangle. You don't want to see that doming any more. If you see it when you lift yourself out of bed or off the floor, make it a habit instead to roll over on to your side and push yourself up with your hands, rather than using your abdominals.

Crunches, sit-ups, planks, leg lowers, etc increase intra-abdominal pressure and therefore place a load down on your pelvic floor or out into your linea alba, so you may see doming or feel heaviness in your pelvic floor when performing them. These should be avoided – *not forever*, but until you've got your breathing and core control firing properly. Heavy lifting increases intra-abdominal pressure, too. If you have a toddler or a small child, chances are you'll be lifting them regularly so you *must* commit to lifting correctly to reduce the load on your pelvic floor (*see* p. 53).

Continue to avoid 'regular' exercises – even if you get the 'all clear to exercise' from the GP at your six-week check-up. Unless they have actually palpated your abdominals to check for DR, please don't rush back into traditional ab exercises, oblique strengtheners (Twisting Curl-ups and Side Planks – *see* p. 175), or twisting movements that feel challenging on the core. Avoid getting back into running or any other high-impact exercise *just yet*. Erring on the side of caution, while keeping active, is always the best policy – despite what some celebrity trainers might suggest on their glossy Instagram feeds.

Excessive abdominal training with a DR, particularly with twisting movements, such as oblique curl-ups, can cause a downward pressure in the abdomen through the pelvic floor, which will pull the already weakened linea alba further out to the sides.

Diastasis recti doesn't always resolve itself on its own. The first eight weeks postnatally are where the main natural healing takes place, and if you still have a problem gap after this point it needs conscious training and dedicated deep core healing work.

Postnatal exercise

The 'bounce back' pressure is so toxic because it offers mums yet another area in which to feel like we're failing. I really do understand how keen you are to get 'back to your pre-baby self'. Body image is so intrinsic to happiness and identity, and postnatally this can take a real beating. There is so much healing going on under the skin, you need nurturing and kindness. If you do go to a Postnatal Boot Camp BODY BACK-type fitness class, your instructor should ideally check your abdominals for separation and *at the very least* ask you about your birth experience and how your pelvic floor is feeling. If the instructor omits any of these essential duty-of-care issues, and particularly if they focus on planking, crunches, 'feeling the burn', burpees, leg lowers, flat tummy exercises etc, please, do not do this class.

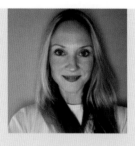

EXPERT ADVICE

I love being a mum. For me it was the most amazing, wonderful (and scary) thing that ever happened to me. I also love to run and as soon as I had my children, on both occasions, I wanted to get out there, clocking up the distance as soon as I could.

However, I am also a women's health physiotherapist and I know just what a life-changing event pregnancy and childbirth is. Your body changes in incredible ways, and the reality is that EVERY woman will have a weaker pelvic floor, glutes, tummy muscles and altered posture. Such a cocktail can lead to urinary/faecal incontinence, pelvic organ prolapse, dyspareunia (pain in the genitals during sex), unresolving diastasis recti and musculoskeletal injuries, i.e. low back pain.

Even if you had the most beautiful, serene pregnancy and childbirth there is no getting away from such physiological changes. Even if you have no symptoms, i.e. urinary incontinence, it does not mean that six weeks post delivery you are ready to return to high-impact/- level exercise. Ladies, we need to think long-term prevention when it comes to postnatal recovery because unless these weaknesses are addressed, at some stage in life pelvic floor dysfunction can occur no matter who you are.

The stumbling block is that there is so much conflicting information out there and we do not receive the level of postnatal rehabilitation we need and deserve. If you had knee surgery you would always see a physiotherapist post op. I advocate that every woman regardless of delivery sees a women's health physiotherapist anytime from six weeks post baby. The six-week GP check is not enough. Many women's health physiotherapists now carry out a 'Mummy MOT'. This involves a musculoskeletal assessment of your back, pelvis, global muscle strength, tummy check and, importantly, an internal assessment of your pelvic floor. From there, a programme is devised to put you on the right track to recovery, bespoke to you and your goals.

Before I returned to running I did just that. I visited a colleague who helped me retrain my pelvic floor and core. I did not return to running until six months after both of my children were born and for the vast majority of this time used Pilates to build up my foundations, which ensured that I could return to running without incurring any pelvic floor dysfunction or musculoskeletal issues.

It takes time to heal and regain your strength, you are only human. There is no shame in prioritising you and getting your body back safely and effectively. If you return to sit-ups, planks, high impact too soon you can do more harm than good. So ladies, please, ask your GP to refer you to a women's health physiotherapist and look after YOU!

Emma (Physiomum) is a specialist women's health physiotherapist, based in Oxted, Surrey. Her particular area of interest is in postnatal rehabilitation and working with women to return to high-impact exercise and running safely and effectively. You can follow her on Instagram: physiomumuk, Facebook: @physiomum.co.uk; or on Twitter @emma_physiomum

THE REC CHECK

Checking for DR is simple, but *ask a professional to check you as well as having a feel for yourself.* A DR gap is measured in finger distance, and can occur at any place along the linea alba. A gap of one to two fingers' width is normal post delivery.

- Lie in Relaxation Position (*see* p. 56), taking one hand behind your head.
- Place three fingers just in the centre of your abdominals, above the navel.
- Palpate (press firmly down) to have a feel of the muscles.
- Gently lift your head and continue to press down, and feel how your muscles react.
- Relax the head down, then slide your leg away, still palpating your abdomen to notice for tension and recruitment of the muscles.

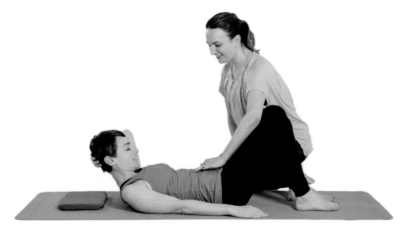

- As you lift your head, connect to your centre: engage your pelvic floor and TA, so that you can have an idea of the *tone* supporting the linea alba. By 'tone' I mean it should feel firm and springy in the space in between the sides of the rectus muscle. Even if there is a significant 'gap' of more than two fingers, the presence of tone indicates that it is *functional*, which is the most important thing.
- If it feels like you're pressing deeply into a soft blancmange without any tension, that's a serious gap that needs to be looked at by a physio; there is a proven link between DR and pelvic floor dysfunction – 66 per cent of women with DR also have a pelvic floor dysfunction (research from 2011 Lee, Hodges, Wiebe), so it's not something to be ignored.

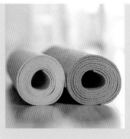

CASE STUDY

Hina, mum of two

I spent a month doing dedicated work on my diastasis recti and I am beyond thrilled that I healed it! I went from being able to put four fingers in the gap to barely being able to push a finger in and clearly feeling the muscle tone. I took guidance and did Pilates every day for about four weeks, and I am so blown away by what happened.

Your ribcage

Your ribcage contains your lungs and your heart. During pregnancy it flares to accommodate your baby, and your diaphragm and lungs are pushed up as your baby expands into the space. Your pregnancy posture may also have made your chest roll forwards, which compresses your breastbone and lungs, and it'll take time to recalibrate. Breathing is so important. Aim for an umbrella breath – opening your lungs out 360 degrees as you breathe in and closing them on the out-breath. This begins to massage the intercostal muscles, in between each rib, to enable full movement of the ribcage.

Imagine a church bell sitting in the centre of your chest. When your ribcage is centred directly above your pelvis, in balance, the bell hangs silent. If you droop forwards, the bell clangs forwards. If you flare your ribcage, the bell clangs back. Take a moment to notice your alignment of your ribcage. Check in the mirror if you can – are you 'ringing up' or 'ringing down'?

To help realign the ribcage with the pelvis, in order to begin to restore abdominal strength and heal diastasis recti, we often need to draw the bottom of the ribcage back in line with the top of the pelvis. Imagine softly hugging your lower ribs back in towards your heart: maintaining height, but drawing your ribs back so that they are in line with the hips. Use your hands: palpate the space between your lower rib and your hip bones.

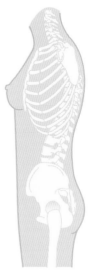

Balanced rib–pelvis connection

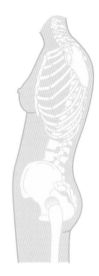

Unbalanced rib-pelvis connection

Your feet

Another common yet surprising issue postnatally is your feet. In whole-body terms, foot problems can often contribute to general weakness and imbalance in the pelvic floor so it's important to be aware of the way that you balance on your feet day to day. During pregnancy, the relaxin hormone affects the ligaments, and this can result in fallen arches. It's therefore important to wear supportive shoes and regularly work on foot stability with balance work: try standing up on your tiptoes slowly and deliberately while the kettle is boiling, lower back down then repeat 10 times. Other good exercises are Pliés (p. 88) and Lunges (*see* p. 178).

Foot exercises are really important. Try these: Imagine playing the piano with your toes, moving each toe individually. Lift your big toes on their own. Lower back down. Lift your little toes. Lower back down. Try to grip and pick up a towel from the floor with your feet. Activities like this stimulate the muscles in your feet, work your arches and massage the connective tissue. When you're standing, send your awareness to your feet, the triangle of connection of your big toe joint, your little toe joint, and your heel. There is a definite link between foot strength and the pelvic floor – if you're able to properly ground through these points in your feet, this has a lifting and supporting effect on your pelvic muscles.

Long term, think about your feet as a starting point for all your posture awareness. Try to make sure you spend at least some time each day in bare feet, literally grounding yourself. Changes in foot stability and stiffness creeps up into your body and affects all of your movement patterns. Rolling your foot on a tennis ball daily is a great way to massage the fascia and encourage good foot – and therefore influence whole-body – function and health.

Plantar fasciitis

Plantar fasciitis – inflammation and tearing in the tissues on the bottom of the foot – is common. It can present as annoying foot or heel pain when standing up after sitting or lying down for a while (such as first thing in the morning, when you might hobble painfully getting out of bed). An easy way to help alleviate inflammation is to put a bottle of water in the freezer, and in the morning roll your foot along it.

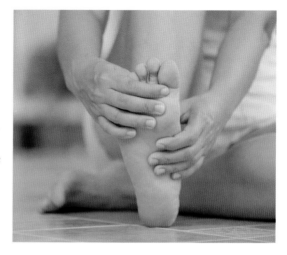

Posture

Posture is such an integral part of our wellbeing, yet we can be completely oblivious to how we carry ourselves. When you think of posture you might think of 'standing or sitting up straight'. But posture isn't 'held' or static: it's responsive, dynamic, constantly recalibrating according to what you're doing (kind of like motherhood itself…).

Posture is the alignment of your skeleton and muscles. It's also reflective of a state of mind: if you feel low, your shoulders will droop, your chest collapses and your heart and lungs are squashed. So many 'mum duties' involve hunching forwards, and over time this can have a cumulative negative impact on your sense of wellbeing and positivity *without you even realising*.

Pilates encourages you to check in with your posture every day, and 'imprint' better posture into your body awareness. Make use of a mirror – or take pictures on your phone or have your partner do so – and really observe the way you carry yourself. You have the power to change your postural habits, and therefore directly influence the way that motherhood challenges your body. When you're standing and pushing your buggy/wearing your baby, check in with your posture often: soften your shoulders, lift up tall through the crown of your head, look up.

'Ideal' standing posture

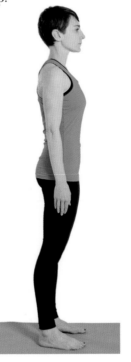
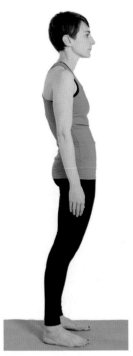

- Your head is lengthened at the top of the spine, not tilted forwards or back.
- Your shoulder blades lie flat against your ribcage.
- The bottom of the ribcage is aligned with the top of your pelvis: not shifted forwards or tucked down, so the lungs have plenty of space for efficient breathing.
- The natural curves of the spine are preserved.
- The pelvis is neutral (*see* p. 55), not tilted forwards or back.
- The knee joints are in line with the hips and ankles.
- The head, ribcage and pelvis are balanced directly over the arch of your foot.

Common mum posture.

Your postnatal posture

Your body balance and centre of gravity changes throughout your pregnancy, and this altered 'map' of your muscles can remain long into motherhood unless actively reconditioned. Often, there's an increased curve in the upper back (kyphosis), which is created by the extra weight of your boobs, not to mention all baby-related activities involving forward hunching, and there is often an increased curve (lordosis) in the neck and in the lumbar spine (lower back) due to the way you carried your baby and the forward tilting of the pelvis that often happens as a result of this.

In some women, during pregnancy the lumbar spine flattens and the pelvis tilts back in the opposite way, switching off the bottom muscles. This can be a common 'mum posture' when you're constantly swinging a small person on to your hip or baby wearing a lot. Your joints and muscles are misaligned and all of your movement patterns are affected, which means aches and pains usually follow. Pilates is ideal for counterbalancing this load on your body, for *noticing* how you carry yourself and consciously deciding to rectify poor posture.

Protecting your back while lifting and carrying your baby/toddler

You need to be mindful of your posture while picking up your baby/ lifting your toddler into the buggy, etc. Lifting your little one in and out of the cot/bath requires conscious stability. The same goes for car seats: they wreak havoc on our backs as they weigh a tonne, and commonly we lift them when we're a bit stressed and being shouted at by a small person, so any mindful movement intention goes out the window.

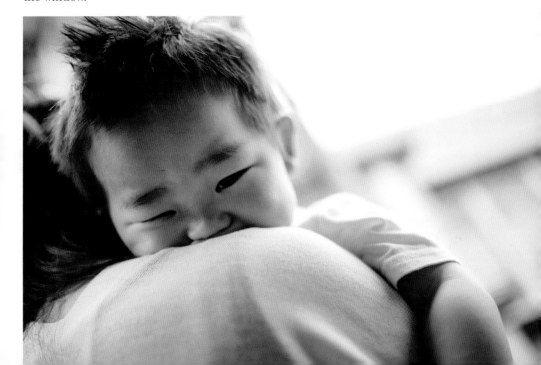

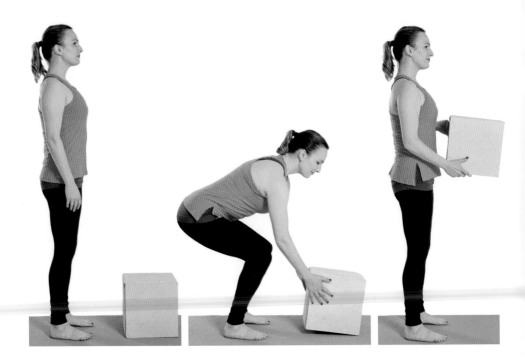

Whenever you bend down to lift or dress your toddler/
child, make sure that you squat down, bending your hips
and knees, rather than hanging your spine forwards with
straight legs. Try to make sure you're standing as close as
possible to your toddler when you pick them up, rather
than reaching for them as they scarper away from you.
When you lift, breathe out and engage your pelvic floor
actively. Be aware of and try to avoid carrying your child
repeatedly on the same side.

As mums, we tend to become pack horses without
blinking: carrying buggies up stairs at stations, walking
home from school carrying your toddler, her scooter, his
trumpet and all your shopping... We pile up our physical
duties without questioning it because we just have to
get things done. This puts us at very real risk of back/
shoulder/neck injury and pain.

Movements that combine twisting with bending (such
as lifting your baby out of the bath) put the most pressure
on the spine, and this is when you're likely to injure
yourself if you're not mindful. Lifting and transporting
a toddler can be a very challenging task, particularly if
they're playing dead, or planking. Always lift with care.
Switch your baby changing bag to a rucksack and make
sure you carry it on your back and not on one shoulder.

Tip

When you lift your child
in and out of their cot/
car seat/bath, connect to
your centre first. Consider it
an active pelvic floor/core
functional exercise, rather
than something you do
without thought. All of my
clients suffering from pelvic
floor and diastasis recti issues
heal faster and see more
progress in their symptoms
when they bring their body
awareness into their daily
movement habits.

ABCs: ALIGNMENT, BREATHING, CENTRING

The Pilates principles that should underpin all your sessions (and movement in life) are the 'ABCs' – alignment, breathing, centring. The following pages are some fundamental exercises suitable for all stages of your postnatal recovery, to lay the groundwork for your Pilates practice.

Alignment

Neutral pelvis and spine

Joe Pilates said, 'If your spine is inflexibly stiff at 30, you are old. If it is completely flexible at 60, you are young.'

The key to maintaining the flexibility (and youth!) of your spine is creating optimum space between your vertebrae, to encourage length within the spine for the intervertebral discs to operate, which preserves their cushioning effect in the long term. Being in a 'neutral' position means that your spine is balanced in its natural curves: there is no compression or unwanted flexion or extension within the spine. Neutral is the optimum position for your spine to withstand the forces of gravity. Your spinal curves are your body's shock absorbers, so if they are slightly out of kilter or continually held out of balance, that affects the way that your body will take the repetitive 'shock' of your daily movement.

Neutral pelvis and spine are interrelated, but not the same thing. Your pelvis can maintain neutral when your spine isn't, for example during Curl-ups (*see* p. 147). Neutral pelvis is when your pelvis is lengthened at the end of your spine, with the hip bones (your ASIS: anterior and superior iliac spine) and pubic bone level with each other. Your tailbone is neither tucked nor arched. If your pelvis isn't in neutral, your lumbar spine will either be flattened or will be arched, in response to the position of the pelvis.

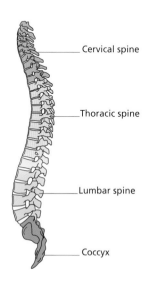

Cervical spine

Thoracic spine

Lumbar spine

Coccyx

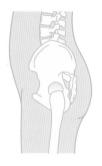

Neutral standing pelvis

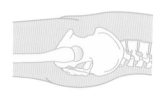

Neutral lying pelvis

RELAXATION POSITION
Stage 1

This exercise prepares you for movement and relaxes your muscles, allowing you to settle into your neutral alignment and breathing. It's also a wonderful way of softening the demands of motherhood: I recommend doing this every single day. You can do it even with your baby lying on you or your toddler climbing over you.

- Lie on your back, arms lengthened down by your sides, or resting your hands on your belly. Feet flat on the floor, knees bent, hip-width apart.

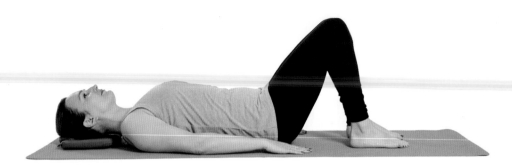

- Lengthen your body. Imagine you're lying on soft sand; consider the imprint that your body would be making. Soften all 10 toes. Imagine the thigh bones dropping into their sockets. Feel the pelvis release heavily into the mat.
- Surrender your weight to the mat without collapsing: allow your position to have intention.
- Travel awareness up the spine: notice your lumbar curve. Is it flat towards the mat, or arched? Place the back of your hand into the small of your back to feel how much space you have there.
- Release the back of your ribcage. Bring a rhythm to your breath: in for a count of five, out for a count of six.
- Relax the shoulders and lengthen your neck. Make sure your face is parallel with the ceiling and your chin isn't higher than your nose, or tucked towards your chest.

FINDING NEUTRAL – PELVIC TILTS
Stage 1

- Place your hands on your belly: connect your thumbs and fingertips to form a diamond shape, with the heels of your hands on your hip bones (bony parts of your pelvis) and your fingertips towards your pubic bone.

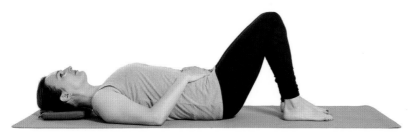

- Imagine your pelvis is a bowl of thick soup. At rest in neutral, the surface of your soup is level. Tuck your tailbone underneath you, tilt the pelvis and imagine the soup slowly tipping towards your belly button. Your lumbar spine releases into the mat, out of its natural curve.

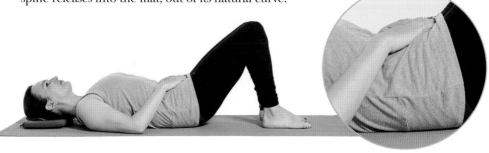

- Send your tailbone away, visualise the soup tipping towards your heels. The lumbar spine is arched out of its natural curve.
- Come to a middle point where the soup is completely level. The pelvis is level. The lumbar spine is in its natural curve. This is neutral.

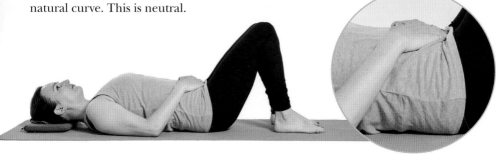

Breathing

Your breath is inextricably linked with your pelvic floor health and postnatal recovery. This might sound dull, but tweaking your breathing and focusing on it on a daily basis will mean that everything slots back into place quicker; it's for this reason that if you visit a women's health physio at this stage, the first session will focus on your alignment and breathing. What's more, it also stimulates your nervous system response, which will calm your mind. This in turn releases tension in your body: a calm mind sends a signal to your body that it's OK to switch off; it's safe to heal.

Deep breathing is also useful if you're trying to establish breastfeeding and it's painful, or you're generally feeling tense and anxious. Breathe out slowly and steadily while you put your baby on the breast, and soften into the discomfort rather than fighting it.

SCARF BREATHING
Stage 1

This exercise encourages you to find your full wide Pilates breath. The scarf gives you a feedback for where your ribcage is: you can feel your lungs opening and the intercostal muscles of your ribcage expanding as the ribcage widens into the scarf. You could also use a stretchy band or a yoga strap instead of a scarf.

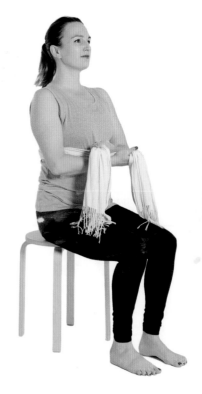

- Sitting or standing, wrap a scarf or band around your lower ribs – just below your bra-strap area. Hold opposite ends of the band/scarf and pull it quite tight so you can feel there is comfortable tension around your ribcage and upper waist.
- As you breathe in, imagine your ribcage expanding to the sides like bellows. Allow the breath to expand into your ribs and then down into the abdomen.
  Try not to overbreathe. Make sure your chest and shoulders stay soft and heavy.
- Sigh the breath out as if you're trying to fog a window in front of you. Your hands should be able to draw the band across your body as the ribcage closes while the lungs empty.

Remember: breathe fully and naturally. If it feels forced, relax and allow it to soften into a more natural pattern. Pilates breathing will become normal with practice.

PISTON BREATH
Stage 1

Julie Wiebe is a physical therapist specialising in women's health and postpartum recovery. She describes the Piston System of the diaphragm, pelvic floor and transversus abdominis (TA) working in conjunction with each other, in balance. The diaphragm is the starting point, needing space to open and perform its function effectively. That in turn creates space for the pelvic floor and TA to activate optimally.

Picture the torso as a cylinder. As you breathe in, visualise the diaphragm, and your pelvic floor and TA descending, like a piston. As you breathe out, the momentum is directly up, with the diaphragm and with the pelvic floor and TA. This is a natural functional momentum. If there is a weakness in the natural momentum, pressure will distend down or the abdominals will brace.

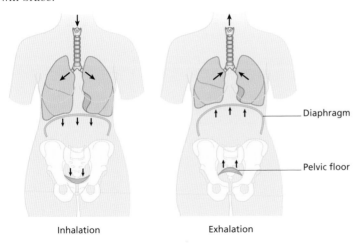

Diaphragm

Pelvic floor

Inhalation   Exhalation

Tip

Take some time to notice your breath. Sit or lie with one hand on your belly, the other on your heart. Allow your hands to 'listen' to your body in stillness for a moment. Notice any movement through your torso with your breath. Allowing your diaphragm to fully descend, your abdomen will expand, and that is *good* – too many of us don't ever release our abdominals, so they become tight and put pressure down into the pelvic floor – *see* Piston Breath, above, and also Sniff, Flop, Drop on p. 99. This is one of the most important ways to begin allowing relaxation and release, and proper function of your abdominal/pelvic muscles.

Centring

Pelvic floor – finding your centre

How should it feel? How do I know if I'm doing it right? Remember **Stage 1** of our postnatal journey. Pelvic floor *awareness* is key. You can't strengthen what you can't connect to.

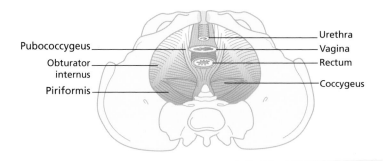

Pubococcygeus

Obturator internus

Piriformis

Urethra

Vagina

Rectum

Coccygeus

Help! I can't feel it!

Scar tissue from birth injury (whether vaginal or Caesarean birth) or overly tense core muscles may affect your awareness, control and sensation of your pelvic floor. So try not to feel frustrated with yourself if it seems impossible to find. It may be that there are physical or emotional factors blocking your connection. Try these tips:

o If you really can't find your pelvic floor at all, try sucking your thumb, blowing on your hand, or coughing. This should trigger your natural pelvic floor lift. Persevere with the pelvic floor *awareness* exercises – it's a subtle sensation, so it may simply be that you need to find that mindful connection to your body, and relax into it. Practise the Pelvic Floor Meditation (*see* p. 182) every day to see if that helps.

o Palpate with your hands – on the outside of your pelvis, or inside your vagina (wash your hands first obviously): it's your body! We're quite squeamish about this part of our anatomy, but we really shouldn't be, particularly after having a baby. Your own touch is very important post episiotomy or stitches to help break down scar tissue and encourage your sensation back. Find and visualise where the muscle attaches: feel your sit bones with your fingers, press your fingers around your pelvis.

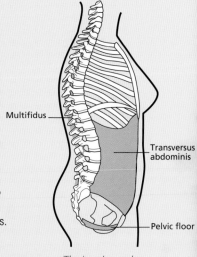

Multifidus

Transversus abdominis

Pelvic floor

The 'core' muscles.

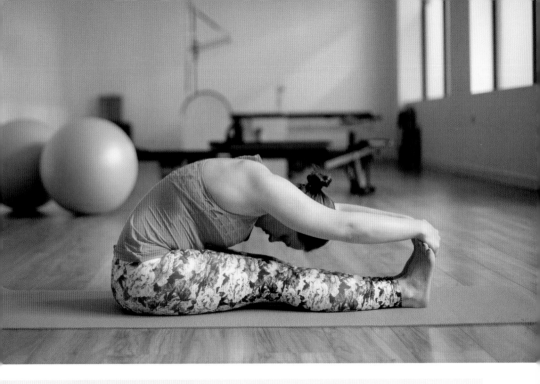

- o Sit forwards a bit with a tall spine and then use your hands to pull your bum cheeks out from underneath you, to make sure you're sitting on your sit bones. Hinge from the hips and lean slightly forwards. Imagine pulling all sides of your pelvic floor together and then up inside you through your vagina. It's a very deep feeling, a bit like pulling up a tampon inside you. Try to pull up slowly, release and repeat 10 times, three times a day, every day. Then, once you've mastered a slow draw-up and hold, then try for 10 quicker 'contract-release, contract-release'. There's a hashtag started by the brilliant women's health physio and stand-up comedian Elaine Miller (@gussetgrippers) #wewontpeewith10103: 10 slow-lift contractions, then 10 quicker contractions, three times a day – this genuinely will make a difference to your pelvic floor health *if you actually do it.*

- o See how it feels to squeeze your finger inside you: if firing correctly, it should feel a bit like a baby sucking on your finger and you should be able to hold this for 5–10 seconds. If you cough, *this squeeze should happen automatically.* Having a tactile approach may help you to mentally connect to the engagement and unlock a physical sensation that was otherwise eluding you.

If you still struggle to connect – and particularly if you've found pelvic floor sensation elusive since your birth(s) or have been suffering from urinary or faecal incontinence – go to a women's health physiotherapist without delay.

PELVIC FLOOR CONNECTION
Stage 1
Here we learn to *soften* to find your centre.

- Sit upright on a chair – or lie down if that helps you connect better. Your feet are hip-width apart, with your weight evenly released into your feet and sit bones.

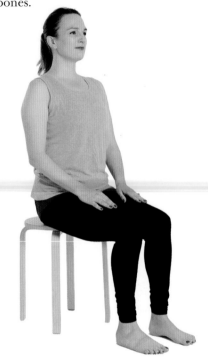

- Sigh your breath out, then lift your back passage, as if you're trying to stop breaking wind. Continue this lifting energy towards your pubic bone. Engage from back to front, up and in. We want to locate the full breadth of the muscles from the back to the front, *and from the sides in.* Imagine a diamond shape: the pubic bone at the front, the two sit bones either side and the tailbone at the back. Visualise the diamond shape drawing in and up from all points.

- Breathe in and let the engagement go: fully release it like dropping a marble into a glass of water.
- Repeat a few times.

Watchpoints
Scan your body for tension. Check that you haven't also tensed your jaw, buttocks, inner thighs or are bracing your upper stomach. It's an *internal,* outwardly invisible engagement. Yes, that includes your eyebrows. Keep them soft.

If you lose your connection, don't feel frustrated. Take a breath and start again. With practice, it will become more natural.

Tip
Don't practise this while sitting on the loo, stopping mid-flow while actually having a pee. That potentially creates bladder dysfunction by disrupting the message that you need to pee. You also might introduce the chance of a urinary tract infection. Please *imagine* stopping the flow of wee rather than actually doing it.

A note about pelvic organ prolapse and daily activities

Do you feel like daily baby duties, such as pushing your buggy, make your pelvic floor symptoms worse? If you have a vaginal prolapse, exertion can feel like it aggravates your prolapse symptoms*. Here are some tips if you're struggling:

o Check your breathing. Are you holding your breath? Instead, try picturing your breath expanding out 360 degrees. On an inhalation, let your ribs expand and your tummy and pelvic floor soften. On the exhalation, allow for a gentle natural lift as you push the buggy up on to the pavement.

o Try a different tension strategy. Are you bracing and squeezing, trying to hold everything in as you exert effort? What happens if you 'let go' a bit?

o Try a change in position. Bring your hips back, or maybe forwards. Drop your ribs down, or broaden your chest. *Can you feel a difference?*

o Try to switch on your buttocks – this will help you to find the power to push. If you aren't feeling your bum 'kick in' naturally, what happens if you actively try to engage your bum so that you can?

o Adopt a growth mindset: 'I haven't yet found the way to symptom-free buggy pushing so I'll keep trying until I do' versus 'This is a disaster, I'll never push my buggy without symptoms'. *Challenge your limiting thoughts.*

Essentially, do something different and see if it helps – this is always preferable to hoping something will magically get better on its own, or ignoring symptoms entirely. Your postnatal healing journey is not always about following set formulae and rules, but increasing your options and finding what works for you.

Always go to a women's health physio if you think you might have a prolapse.

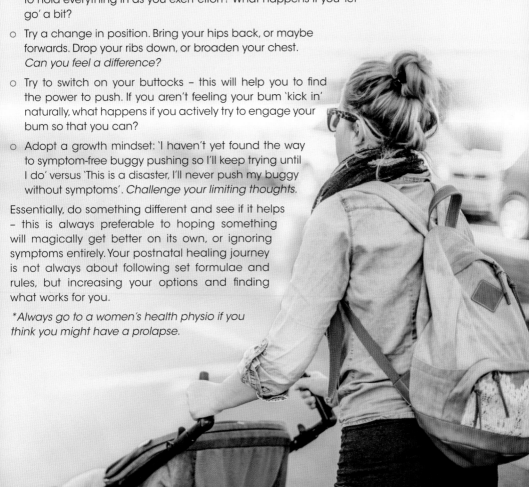

PILATES TO BALANCE YOUR POSTNATAL BODY

Here are some key Pilates exercises that are perfect for the postnatal body. Master these, and you'll be rebalancing your body and strengthening your core beautifully.

WALL POSTURE CHECK AND SIDE REACH
Stage 1

An easy one to build into your day to day as we are usually quite near a wall, and you can do this while making a cup of tea. Builds your general awareness of your posture, and stretches your spine, alleviating tension around the hips and pelvis.

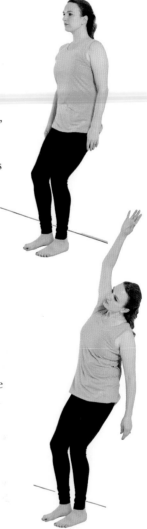

- Stand with your back against a wall. Place your feet a comfortable distance away: about 30cm (12in) as a guide (but make sure it's the right distance for your body proportions). The knees should be able to soften comfortably, directly above your ankles.

- Scan your natural posture. Is your head touching the wall? If not, don't force it, just notice. In an ideal posture, the head lengthens upright away from the shoulder blades and therefore would be in contact with the wall, but in normal life we spend a lot of time stooped and this ideal alignment becomes more unnatural.

- Notice your upper spine. Can you feel your shoulder blades release into the wall? Can you feel the whole of the back of the ribcage or just part of it?

- Notice your lumbar spine. Is there a big gap away from the wall between your bottom and your shoulders, or are you almost flat against it? You can take your hand behind the small of your back and notice if you can thread your hand through the gap completely, or only slightly.

- Think about your pelvis. Is it level or tilted? Can you feel your sacrum (the 'flat' part of your pelvis) releasing back into the wall?

- Breathe in to float one arm out by your side, reaching the arm above your head.

- Breathe out to carry the arm across and lean on the diagonal. Maintain a connection with the wall with both shoulder blades.

- Breathe in to lengthen into the side stretch. Press your hips slightly in the opposite direction to increase the stretch in the side, if that feels OK to you.

- Breathe out to return to centre. Repeat on each side up to 5 times.

BACK STRETCH USING THE WALL/BUGGY

Stage 1

What mums need above all else is to stretch out, like a cat. You can do this stretch using a wall/counter top/buggy bar. It stretches your lower back and hamstrings, lengthens your waist, softens your shoulders and encourages you to breathe deeply and check in with your abdominal connection.

- Standing tall, at arms' length away from the wall, place your palms flat against the wall/resting on the counter top/buggy bar.
- Send your bottom back so that your spine and arms are in one long line.
- Reach the arms away from the tailbone, keeping the neck in line with the spine – don't collapse the head to look into your belly. Look down at the floor.
- Breathe slowly and deeply as you lengthen into the position. Allow your belly to soften, or draw it consciously in – experiment between the two to enhance your awareness of your centre engagement.
- With control, slowly restack your spine to upright.

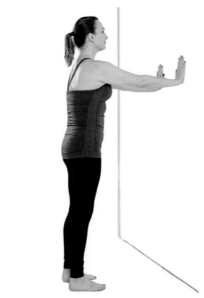

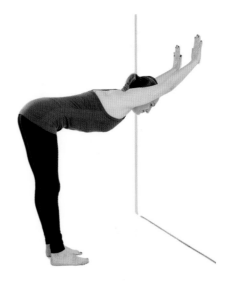

SHOULDER STRETCH

Stage 1

We all suffer from shoulder tension, generally. Add mother duties to the mix – nappies, buggies, endlessly picking up toys and socks, continually holding your baby/toddler on one side – and you're much more likely to hunch forwards. This is a blissful way of stretching out, massaging and mobilising your upper (thoracic) spine. It's a great posture check on the go.

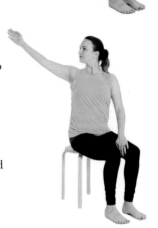

- You can do this standing or sitting. Take the hands on to the shoulders. Bring the elbows together. Imagine the collarbones are wide and open.

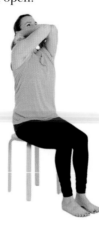

- Breathing normally, keep the elbows together and roll them up towards the ceiling. Allow your eye focus and nose to follow their trajectory and open your chest to the ceiling.

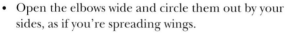

- Open the elbows wide and circle them out by your sides, as if you're spreading wings.
- Bring the elbows back together and allow your head to restack on the top of the vertebrae of your spine.
- Repeat up to 5 times, then reverse the direction.

- Release one arm down and place the palm down on your inner thigh. Keep the other on the shoulder.

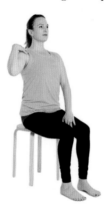

- Open your chest out to the side, then extend your arm up and away.
- Repeat up to 3 times. Breathe deeply and keep the lumbar spine lengthened, not tucked or arching.

SHOULDER STRETCH AGAINST THE WALL
Stage 1

This is a really amazing stretch, particularly for the first few months postnatally, although three years postnatal with my second, I still do this most days. It's a must for opening the chest and releasing tension from buggy stoop. Be gentle with this if you are breastfeeding as the pull on your chest might make your boobs feel tender.

- Stand against a wall, side on. Place your hand on to the wall and then walk it up to shoulder height, then a little bit higher.

- Placing gentle pressure into the wall, keeping the arm softly bent, reach the fingertips away. You can lengthen the arm either in line with your shoulder, or reach higher in a diagonal – whichever feels better for your shoulder joint. Rotate as far as you can feel a stretch into the front of the chest/armpit. Breathe into the stretch.

- If it feels nice, and the mobility is available to you, you can add a full Arm Circle.

- Release your arm and then repeat on the other side.

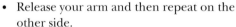

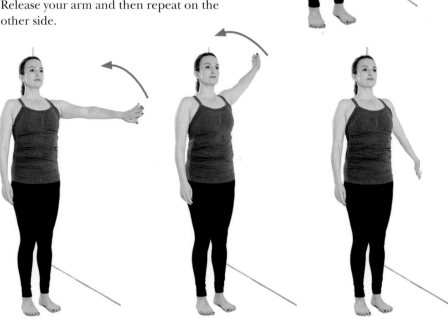

PELVIC STABILITY

The following exercises are great ways of enhancing your core stability and building deep inner strength by introducing movement of the limbs to challenge your control of your pelvis.

LEG SLIDES

Stage 1

In Relaxation Position (*see* p. 56), you could rest your hands on your belly, to check for any movement of your pelvis. You can also do this with the ball underneath your pelvis, as for Compass (*see* p. 75), for extra challenge and feedback.

- Breathe in, lengthen your spine.

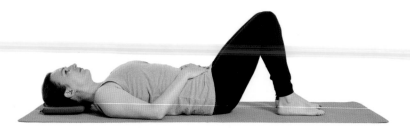

- Breathe out, stabilise and slide one leg along the floor, in line with your hip. Maintain your neutral pelvis and spine.

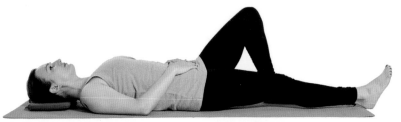

- Breathe in wide, stay active in your centre and return your leg to the start position.

Watchpoint

Make sure your pelvis and spine remain stable and heavy throughout; no rocking.

KNEE DROPS
Stage 1

Really concentrate on the quality of your movement with this exercise: notice whether your pelvis moves and see whether you can develop the strength and control to ensure your pelvis stays stable as you move the thighbones in their sockets.

- Start as for Leg Slides on previous page. Breathe in to prepare, stabilise. You may find that you need to 'turn up' your engagement appropriately, to control the movement.

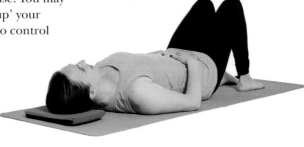

- Breathe out and open one leg out to the side, allowing the foot to roll on to its side. Open the knee as far as you can without disturbing the pelvis. The hip bones (bony parts at the front of your pelvis) should remain parallel with the floor.

- Breathe in to return the leg back to centre.
- Repeat up to 5 times on either side.

Watchpoints

Control the movement. Try to avoid letting the stable leg wander out to the opposite side.

Imagine your hip bones are headlights: they should stay shining up to the ceiling as you move the thighbone away from the body, not travel in the direction of the leg.

If it helps, you can bring your hands underneath your buttocks, palms down. Repeat the exercise and notice if you're sinking your bottom into one hand as you open the leg. See whether you can connect to your centre to ensure you distribute the weight evenly through each side of the pelvis, even when moving the leg challenges this stability. *This is core control.*

BAND PULL WITH KNEE DROP
Stage 2

This exercise challenges your coordination and core strength. The opposite arm and leg movement creates a diagonal engagement across your torso from shoulder to opposite hip – Body Control Pilates® calls it the 'X factor' – which requires deep abdominal strength to keep you stable. Great for rehab for diastasis recti, it's a low-impact, supported way of getting those abdominals working once more.

- Start lying in Relaxation Position (*see* p. 56). Hold a band or a scarf in both hands. Raise both arms up above the shoulder joints, with tension in the band.
- Breathe in to lengthen the spine.

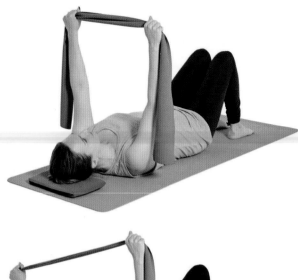

- As you breathe out, open your left arm to the side, pulling the band, but keeping the right arm stable. At the same time, open your right knee out, keeping the pelvis stable.

- Breathe in to return to centre.
- Repeat up to 10 times on each side.
- You can also add Single Knee Folds (*see* p. 71) and Leg Slides (*see* p. 68) to the arm pull.

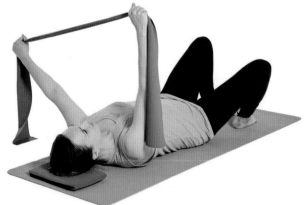

Watchpoints

Keep your pelvis stable and collarbones wide.

Keep the arm straight; try not to bend at the elbow or wrist as you open the band.

SINGLE KNEE FOLDS WITH PELVIC FLOOR WORK
Stage 2

This requires abdominal control. Keep in mind your neutral pelvis throughout.

- Lie in Relaxation Position

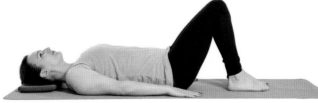

- On an out-breath, float one of your knees towards your chest. Maintain the angle at the knee; try not to let the heel slump towards your bottom. Let the thigh bone drop into its socket, but not so far that the thigh flops into the chest. The shin is parallel with the floor. Your pelvis remains neutral, tailbone heavy. If it feels too easy and there's no effort at all, you're probably cheating.

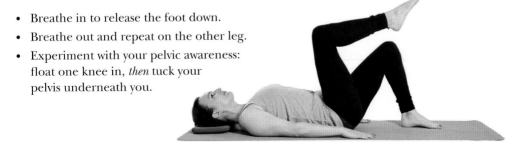

- Breathe in to release the foot down.
- Breathe out and repeat on the other leg.
- Experiment with your pelvic awareness: float one knee in, *then* tuck your pelvis underneath you.

- Using your core control, release your tailbone away from you.
- The thigh bone will move with the pelvis.

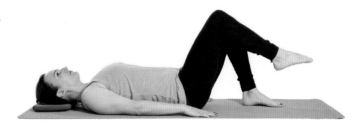

▶

- Return back to neutral.

- Next, place your hand against the thigh. Breathe in to lengthen.

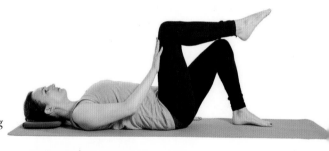

- As you breathe out, press your thigh into your hand and your hand into your thigh – as if you're pushing with equal pressure from both sides. Engage your pelvic floor and lower abdominals strongly as you push.

- Breathe in and release the pressure. Relax. Repeat up to 5 times.

Watchpoints

Fold the knee in line with the hip, not out to the side or across the body.

When pushing into your thigh/hand, ensure that you're not bracing anywhere else in your body. You should feel that your core is active and strong, but everywhere else is relaxed.

OYSTER
Stage 2

This exercise targets your deep gluteal muscles: such important stabilisers of the pelvis and the number one area that mums generally need to strengthen.

- Side-lying, take your feet in line with your bottom, lined up against the side of the mat. Place your top hand in front of your chest, palm down. Or, you may prefer to have your top hand resting on your top hip bone so that you can check for any movement of the pelvis.

- Breathe in, lengthen your spine.

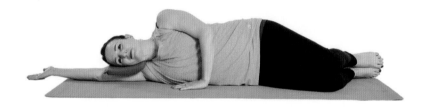

- Breathe out and engage your buttock muscle to open the top knee. Imagine turning your thighbone in its socket like a key in a lock. Keep the feet connected, pressing towards each other like magnets. Your pelvis remains stable and upright. Breathe in and return the knee back to the start position. Imagine you're working under water – there is *resistance* in the movement.

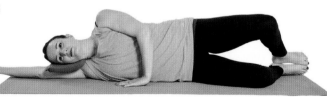

- Repeat up to 10 times, then change sides.

VARIATION
Stage 3

To add a bit more challenge to your stability and really find those deep gluteal muscles, lift the leg to hip height.

- Breathe out and turn out the leg in the same way, but with the leg lifted.

- Breathe in and rotate the thighbone the other way, turning the knee down towards the bottom leg.

- Repeat up to 5 times, then lower the leg back down.

Watchpoints

If you can't feel this in your bum, don't worry – bottoms are renowned for being lazy and hip muscles easily take over. Tip your pelvis slightly *forwards* to make sure your hip muscles aren't working too hard, then try again. You should feel the bum working harder from this angle.

Only go as far as you can keep the pelvis still: the thigh moves independently of the pelvis.

RIBCAGE CLOSURE
Stage 1

Shoulders can get very tight, which can lead to neck and shoulder pain. Your ribcage flares during pregnancy to accommodate your baby growing higher within your torso. Postnatally we need to gently reset our postural patterns and be able to soften the ribs back to their pre-pregnancy position, to help to re-establish good breathing and optimum pelvic floor function. This exercise shows you how to isolate the movement of your shoulders from your torso, connect to your abdominals and become more aware of the stability of your ribcage. You can also do this with a band/scarf, as for ribcage closure with leg slides on page 132.

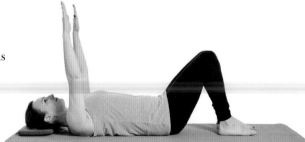

- Begin in Relaxation Position (*see* p. 56).

- Breathe in and raise both arms up towards the ceiling, palms facing forwards.

- As you breathe out, reach both arms back behind you. Maintain a space between your shoulders and your ears. Feel the back of the ribs melting down towards the mat, rather than rising up away.

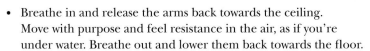

- Breathe in and release the arms back towards the ceiling. Move with purpose and feel resistance in the air, as if you're under water. Breathe out and lower them back towards the floor.
- Repeat up to 10 times.

Watchpoints

Only take your arms back in line with your ears.

Avoid arching the back as shown here: soften the ribs so that they don't 'follow' the arms.

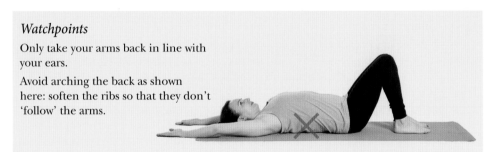

COMPASS

Stage 1

This exercise helps you to build awareness of your pelvic area and is great for gently building pelvic floor strength, stretching your hip flexor muscles and releasing tension in your back. You can also do this with a small Pilates ball underneath your pelvis for feedback.

- Start in Relaxation Position (*see* p. 56). Your lower belly is a compass. Your navel is north, your pubic bone is south and your hip bones on either side are east and west. Breathe in, lengthen the spine.

- Breathe out and tuck your tailbone underneath you, then tilt the pelvis to north, releasing the lumbar spine into the mat.

- Breathe in and roll towards south. The pubic bone moves away from your nose, tilting your pelvis forwards to allow the lumbar spine to softly arch.

- Breathing naturally, repeat this north–south movement a few times.
- Come back to neutral and relax the shoulders and hips. Breathe in to lengthen and prepare.
- Breathe out and this time, roll your pelvis across to east. The opposite buttock will slightly lift off the mat. Keep the feet heavy on the floor.

▶

- Breathe in and roll across to the other side, softening your weight on to the other hip, rolling the pelvis to west.

- Repeat a few times. Become aware of when your pelvis is tilted and when it's in a neutral position.

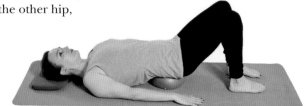

Watchpoints

Keep the knees still and the ribcage and shoulders heavy. Isolate the movement in the pelvis.

Keep the waist long. Imagine you have a mirror above you: your torso remains at the same placement on the mat; it's a pelvic rotation only so there should be no shortening of the waist.

Imagine your pelvis moving around your thigh bones, rather than letting the thigh bones move from side to side. This is a great way of oiling the hip joint.

Check that you're not moving too far south and uncomfortably arching the back.

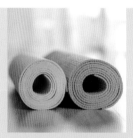

CASE STUDY

Ella, mum of one

If I'm honest, I was in a state of physical and emotional shock after giving birth. I was really lucky to have a straightforward, natural, vaginal delivery but I remember feeling utterly traumatised by how broken my body felt after a three-day labour. I had done NCT classes and remember the NCT teacher saying that the first wee after labour would hurt but after that everything 'down there' would feel normal again… For me it took a good six months for things to feel anywhere near normal.

At three months postpartum I was diagnosed with a grade one uterine prolapse. The fact that this could happen to me, when I was young, healthy, not overweight and active both before and during pregnancy, was a total shock.

Pilates and women's health physio really helped my recovery. I started going to a postnatal Pilates class about five months after the birth and I feel like I only really started to heal my body properly after discovering Pilates

I have had several 'aha moments' during Pilates when I suddenly understood how to correctly engage my deep core and pelvic floor muscles; after months of *thinking* I was doing it right I realised actually I hadn't been. In fact, I think Pilates has helped enhance my understanding of my entire body.

CENTRING IN FOUR-POINT KNEELING
Stage 1

This is one of the best positions to achieve deep lower abdominal recruitment, engaging your stabilising muscles without moving your spine. You spend a lot of time on all fours with babies and toddlers, so this gives you a way of making it a strengthening activity, checking in with how you carry yourself in your normal movement.

- Place your hands directly underneath your shoulders, your knees directly underneath your hips.

- Imagine you're looking at your reflection in a mirror in front of you and lengthen the space from your nose to your breastbone, your breastbone to your navel, your navel to your pubic bone. Take care not to nod your head towards your reflection. If there were a pole placed on your back it would be in contact with your head, mid-back and pelvis.

- Reach the crown of your head forwards and the tailbone back in opposition.

- Try to release into the natural curves of your back. Imagine a friendly cat could curl up in the lumbar curve, but make sure you are not collapsing into an arch. Soften the shoulder blades and lengthen your neck, as if you're a tortoise pushing its head out of its shell.

- Breathe in, allow your abdominals to soften and release. Make sure you don't let the spine drop; stay lengthened.

- Breathe out and draw in from the back passage, bringing this engagement towards your pubic bone. Feel your belly lifting gently in, softening the lower rib towards the top of the pelvis but without moving the spine. Make sure there is no tucking of your pelvis. Think back to your reflection in front of you: the distances should remain even and the torso long.

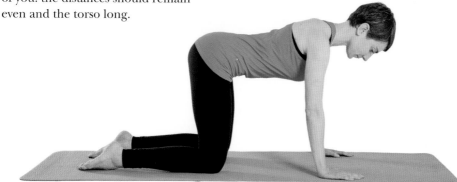

PRONE LEG CIRCLES
Stage 2

This exercise opens the hip joint by working the gluteal muscles (buttocks). It encourages you to find mobility in the hip while keeping the pelvis stable.

- Lying on your front, rest your forehead on a pillow. Your legs are in parallel and hip-width apart. Place your fingertips underneath your hip bones. Feel the pressure that your body weight releases on to your hands. Through this exercise we are aiming to have the pressure stay level on both hands rather than dip into one hand more strongly than the other with the movement. It will take practice! If it's uncomfortable, take your hands up in line with your head, palms down, with your forehead on your hands.
- Breathe in to lengthen the spine.

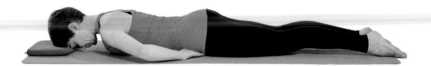

- Breathe out and draw in to your centre. Lengthen and lift one leg away from the floor, opening the hip. Imagine reaching your leg long, towards the wall, away rather than high. You should feel the pressure on that hand remains the same and your lower spine stays soft.
- Draw into your centre. Circle the thighbone 6 times in one direction, then change direction. Feel the movement coming from the top of the thigh, the bottom and hip.

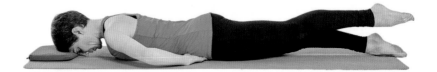

- Breathe in to release back down.
- Repeat up to 3 times on each leg.

Watchpoints

Only lift the leg as high as you can without disturbing the pelvis and arching the back.

Try not to circle from the knee or ankle. Reach out from the hip and feel the buttock muscles fire up.

MOVEMENTS OF THE SPINE

A good Pilates session, however short, will incorporate all movements of the spine. This is to equip you well for your functional daily movement, such as when you're getting up off the floor 300 times a day with baby-related tasks. In each workout, try to balance your body with some flexion (forward bending), extension (backward bending), lateral flexion (sideways bending) and rotation (twisting).

Spinal flexion

Pilates works on fluid sequential movement of the spine, each vertebra moving evenly and independently, like a string of pearls or a bicycle chain. Flexion is the forward rolling movement of the spine.

ROLL-DOWNS AGAINST THE WALL

Stage 2

Mobilise your spine, release tension and wake up your abdominals.

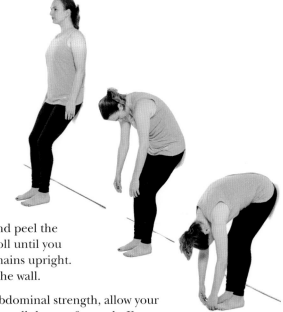

- Stand against the wall. Release your spine fully into the wall, allowing for your natural curve to lengthen, with your feet a comfortable distance away, knees softly bent.

- Breathe in. Lengthen the back of your neck, look down your nose and nod your chin.

- Breathe out, roll your spine forwards, soften your breastbone and peel the spine off the wall, bone by bone. Roll until you reach a point where your pelvis remains upright. Keep your bottom relaxed against the wall.

- If you wish, and feel you have the abdominal strength, allow your hips to hinge now and roll your spine all the way forwards. Keep the knees softly bent. Breathe in, soften your head and arms and relax your neck.

- Breathe out, lengthen the tailbone and unfurl the spine, wheeling back up against the wall, bone by bone. Release the ribcage against the wall, lengthen the head back on top of the spine.

- Repeat up to 5 times.

Watchpoints

Spread your weight evenly on your feet.

Try not to rush. When you rebuild, your head is the last thing to restack on top of your vertebrae.

Completely relax the neck and shoulders, allow them to hang towards the floor like a ragdoll.

CAT-COW
Stages 1-2

This is a great one to do at the end of a chaotic mothering day to soothe your system. And if you are feeling low or depressed, tapping into a feeling of strength by pushing actively into the floor with your hands can ground you and be a way of finding a sense of power.

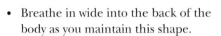

- Begin in Four-point Kneeling (*see* p. 77).

- Breathe in to prepare and lengthen your spine.
- Breathe out and begin to send your tailbone through your legs, rolling the pelvis. Ripple the movement evenly through the spine, flexing each bone away from the one before it. Roll through the hips, the waist, the ribcage, then finally nod the chin softly towards your chest. It's an even flexion of each section of the spine, creating a rainbow 'C-curve' shape.

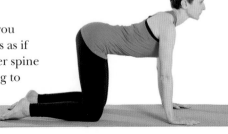

- Breathe in wide into the back of the body as you maintain this shape.
- Breathe out and begin to lengthen the tailbone away from the crown of the head to open the front of your body back to a neutral position.
- Breathe in and lengthen your spine, and as you breathe out, allow the chest to open forwards as if you're shining your heart forwards. The lower spine is supported and not collapsed: you are trying to extend into the *upper* back.
- Repeat up to 10 times, then press yourself back into Rest Position (*see* p. 81).

Watchpoints

Your body will *want to* press up into the ribcage area and fully hunch, which feels really satisfying: but try to focus more on the tuck of the pelvis, full flexion of the lumbar spine. Allow it to be a smooth, even curve throughout.

Make sure your shoulders aren't hunched towards your ears.

Check that your arms aren't locked: the soft part of your elbows should be facing towards each other, not to the front.

Make sure as you shine your heart forwards that you don't overextend your neck: feel a soft pull forwards from the breastbone and allow the neck to stay aligned with your ribs.

REST POSITION
Stage 1

This position stretches the back, nourishes your internal organs and encourages your breath into the back of your body. Perfect for mums for two seconds' peace. Releasing the forehead down is a lovely way to trigger your 'rest and digest' system. It's also an easy way to turn yourself into a climbing frame 'rock' for your little ones while you take five deep breaths...

- Start in Four-point Kneeling.

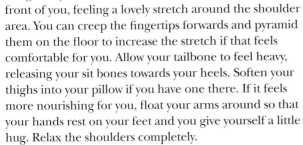

- Breathe in and lengthen the spine.
- Breathe out, release your bottom back towards your heels, hinging at the hips. Lengthen your arms out in front of you, feeling a lovely stretch around the shoulder area. You can creep the fingertips forwards and pyramid them on the floor to increase the stretch if that feels comfortable for you. Allow your tailbone to feel heavy, releasing your sit bones towards your heels. Soften your thighs into your pillow if you have one there. If it feels more nourishing for you, float your arms around so that your hands rest on your feet and you give yourself a little hug. Relax the shoulders completely.
- Allow the forehead to soften into the mat, or on to a pillow. Relax your neck completely.
- Breathe in and allow the breath to travel all the way down your spine towards your pelvis. Relax your belly.

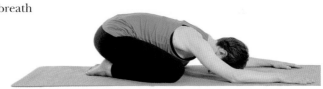

- Keep breathing here for a few breaths, allowing your bottom to release down more heavily with each breath.
- Gradually draw more energy into your centre and as you breathe out, slowly roll back up to sitting, releasing your bottom back onto your heels as you restack the vertebrae of your spine back to upright. Be careful not to come up too quickly, as you'll get a head rush.

SPINE CURLS
Stage 2

This exercise irons out your spine and releases compression, offering you meditative space for breathing. Place a small ball between your knees for a bit more connection to your centre.

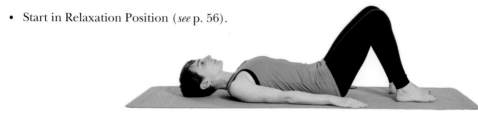

- Start in Relaxation Position (*see* p. 56).

- Breathe in. Lengthen your spine.
- Breathe out and roll your tailbone underneath you, releasing the lumbar spine into the mat. From there, press your feet into the floor as you peel your spine bone by bone, rolling evenly like a bicycle chain, until you reach the bottom of your shoulder blades – or slightly lower.

- Breathe in, sending the knees away over the toes.
- Breathe out, soften your breastbone and release your spine back down, keeping your buttocks lifted and pelvis tucked under until you reach the floor.
- Breathe in to let go of any tension in the shoulders and hips, before repeating on the out-breath.
- Repeat up to 10 times.

Watchpoints

Keep your feet heavy.

Try to find an even sequential movement of your spine: make sure you're not bridging up through any sections as shown here.

Maintain an active connection in the front of your body: soften your bottom rib down into the body as if you're tucking your top into your trousers. Imagine your ribs are connected to your hips with elastic bands: you want the bands to stay taut, not stretched too far.

BRIDGE WITH DOUBLE KNEE DROP
Stage 2

The beauty of this exercise is that we're working in a 'closed chain', whereby your feet and arms are supported by the floor, so there is never too much load going through the pelvis or pressure on your abdominals, but it still really works your core. It also strengthens your buttocks, and challenges your pelvic stability. Be cautious with this variation if you're still suffering from pelvic girdle pain (PGP).

- Start in Relaxation Position (*see* p. 56). Breathe in to prepare your body for movement and lengthen the spine.
- As you breathe out, press the hips and spine in one connected unit up off the mat, hinging from the hips, *not* rolling sequentially as for a Spine Curl (*see* p. 82). Ensure that your spine doesn't arch, squeeze your glutes and soften your ribs.

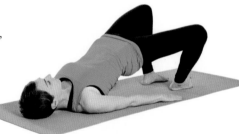

- Breathe in to lengthen, relaxing your shoulders.

- Breathe out, and keeping the bottom lifted, open your right knee to the side, without allowing the right hip to dip. Keep the pelvis stable as if resting on a shelf. Breathe in to stay lengthened.

- Breathe out and open the other knee. Breathe in to lengthen the spine.
- Breathe out to bring the first knee back in, followed by the second. Then, as you breathe in lower the hips down in one go, with the knees apart.

- Push the hips back up on your out-breath. The knees are apart, like 'frog's legs'.

  Repeat 5 times, then bring one leg back to centre followed by the second, then lower the spine down with control.

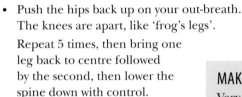

MAKE IT HARDER
Vary the challenge by slowing down your movement, or making it quicker.

SPINAL EXTENSION

Extension is essential for strengthening the back muscles to counterbalance the motherhunch that all baby duties encourage: changing nappies, pushing buggies, feeding, scrolling on your phone... Small babies should be placed on their front regularly so that they develop these back muscles and create strength for movement – they'll never learn to crawl if they aren't placed on their front regularly – and good upright posture. Tummy time is just as essential for mums!

DART
Stage 2

The perfect mum-stoop antidote, this targets those mid-back muscles that are so important for good posture.

- Lie on your tummy. Rest your forehead on a folded towel, or a small flat cushion. Release your arms down by your sides, palms facing up. Your legs are relaxed with your toes together and heels releasing apart. Breathe in to lengthen and prepare.

- Breathe out. Initiate the movement first with your head lengthening away from your spine. Feel your chest open and shoulder blades drawing down on your ribcage, as you begin to peel your chest away from the floor. Stay in contact with the mat with your lower ribs. Your eye focus is down. Lift your arms to reach down by your sides, rotating them so that your palms now face the floor and your shoulder blades draw towards each other. Simultaneously, connect your heels together, engaging your inner thighs to bring your legs into parallel.

- Breathe in and lengthen the spine to maintain this long dart shape, reaching the crown of your head away from your toes.

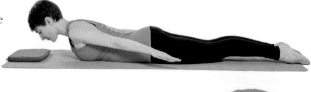

- Breathe out and release your chest, head and arms back to the floor with control. Soften the legs open.
- Repeat up to 10 times, then release back into Rest Position (*see* p. 81).

Watchpoints

Your eye focus stays down towards the floor, neck long and in line with your upper back.

Feel this in the mid-back postural muscles, around the bra strap area, *not* lower, in your lumbar spine. Stay low and long to avoid compressing your lower back.

SPINAL ROTATION

Your ribcage is an area prone to stiffness, pain and tension throughout pregnancy and into motherhood. Twisting movements will help to alleviate some of this and keep the whole spine and the systems of your body balanced, healthy and functioning well. It's so important for your postnatal recovery to encourage your breath wide into the ribcage to help stimulate optimum pelvic floor function.

Twisting is also the movement that you'll do 73,000 times a day lifting your baby out of their cot or bath, or placing your toddler in the car seat (i.e. twisting while carrying a heavy weight), so it's very important to make sure you're mobile and strong enough not to injure yourself in these daily movements. Having badly injured my knee simply by standing up from crouching with my baby in the sling, I know how frustrating and pointless (yet common) that scenario is.

CHALK CIRCLES
Stages 1–2

This is a soothing exercise, supporting controlled mobilisation of the spine, stretching the chest, requiring fluid movements of the shoulder joint with rotation of the spine. It massages your internal organs, encouraging space within your torso. The perfect Pilates exercise for mums.

- Lie on your side. Place a cushion or small ball in between your knees. Make sure your head is in line with your spine: a couple of flat pillows or one bigger cushion should be fine. Lengthen your arms out in front of you, palm on top of palm.
- Breathe in and travel the top arm along the floor, up above your head. Rotate the head in line with the palm.

- Breathe out as you continue to move the hand above your head, drawing a circle along the mat or hovered slightly above. Open the chest to roll the spine back, allowing the arm to open back behind you. Keep looking towards your hand. The hips, knees and ankles remain stacked and still.

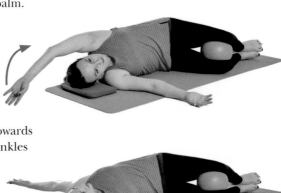

- Circle the arm back down towards your hip and then back to the start position.
- Repeat up to 8 times.

VARIATION

Stage 2

Add a leg extension to give a lush opening to the side of the body and add a bit more challenge to your strength and coordination.

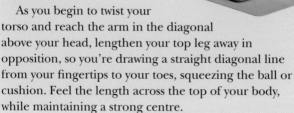

As you begin to twist your torso and reach the arm in the diagonal above your head, lengthen your top leg away in opposition, so you're drawing a straight diagonal line from your fingertips to your toes, squeezing the ball or cushion. Feel the length across the top of your body, while maintaining a strong centre.

Watchpoints

Make sure the movement comes from your torso twisting, not just from the arm reaching back. Only roll as far as you can maintain eye contact with your palm, as though your nose and your middle finger were connected by a puppet string.

Relax the shoulder away from your chin: there should be a space between the neck and the shoulder.

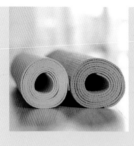

CASE STUDY

Elizabeth, mum of two, postnatal PT and doula
@themummycoach.co.uk

In the months that followed my second child's birth, with a toddler and a newborn to care for, I didn't have much time or energy for exercise. For many months my routine focused solely on Pilates. I'm a runner and used to high-impact exercise so at first I found it slow and strange. It took me right back to basics, forcing me to focus on my breathing and posture and helping me to restore a solid foundation. I loved the fact that I could practise without leaving the house and didn't need masses of equipment. Pilates truly felt like it nourished my post-baby body from deep within.

HIP ROLLS
Stage 2

This is a feel-good twisting exercise. Use your core muscles to roll with control, rather than using the momentum of rolling the legs from side to side. This exercise targets the oblique abdominals in the waist, and the inner thighs. If you have diastasis recti, be cautious of doing too many reps of this: overworking the oblique muscles places a pull on the linea alba, so build it up slowly, focusing on your deep core engagement. This version adds a much-needed chest opener by having the arms lengthened above your head in a Y shape – but if this is tricky for your shoulders or feels in any way uncomfortable across the upper body, bolster your arms with pillows or have the arms released down by your sides in a low upside down V (**Stage 1**).

- Lie in Relaxation Position (*see* p. 56), with your knees and feet connected: imagine you're holding a diamond between your knees and you don't want anyone to steal it. You can squeeze a pillow or small ball between your knees if it helps you to maintain the connection. Reach your arms up to the ceiling and lengthen them behind you, released on the floor in a wide Y shape. Palms up.

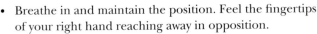

- Breathe in, lengthen the spine.
- Breathe out. Keeping the legs connected, roll your pelvis to the left, rolling your knees to the left. The right side of your bottom will lift as you roll. Keep the feet moving together – they will peel off the mat as the body rotates. The spine moves sequentially: pelvis, waist, ribcage, as for a Spine Curl (*see* p. 82).

- Breathe in and maintain the position. Feel the fingertips of your right hand reaching away in opposition.
- Breathe out, then 'turn up the brightness' of your centre to return your spine and knees back to the start position with control.
- Repeat on the other side, and to each side 5 times.

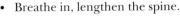

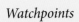

> ### Watchpoints
> Keep your waist long.
>
> Soften the bottom rib towards the top of the pelvis, to ensure you're not arching your back.
>
> Keep your legs connected into your centre: try not to let them 'hang' off the pelvis without control.

LATERAL FLEXION

Involving side reaching, lengthening the waist and rolling the vertebrae of the spine to the side, lateral flexion is so important for mums to stretch tight hips and even out the body.

PLIÉS WITH SIDE REACH
Stage 2

A double boost – work on your buttock strength and ankle-knee-hip alignment, while at the same time doing a fabulous side stretch to open up your waist, challenge your balance a bit and release tension.

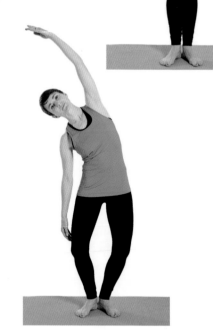

- Begin in Pilates Stance: stand tall, with your heels connected and your toes hip-width apart. 'Zip up' your connection between your inner thighs and gluteal muscles, as if you're wearing a tight pencil skirt. Lengthen your spine and release your arms down by your side.

- Breathe out and bend the knees directly over your toes, into Plié. At the same time, lengthen your left arm up and out to the side and begin to bend your upper body over in a diagonal to the right. Only go as far as you can keep the pelvis square.

- Breathe in to return to the centre, straighten the legs and lower the arm down. If you wish to add further challenge, keeping the heels and thighs working together, rise up onto your toes then release the heels back down.

- Repeat to the other side. Repeat up to 10 times in each direction.

Watchpoints

Ensure your spine doesn't bend forwards, or twist. This should be a purely sideways reach.

Stay lifted in the supporting side of your waist, lengthening evenly in a diagonal as if between two panes of glass.

UPRIGHT HIP FLEXOR SIDE REACH
Stage 2

This is a wonderful stretch that is slightly challenging for your core as it requires balance and stability, so stick with the lying version of Hip Flexor Stretch (*see* p. 109) in the next chapter if you feel any niggling in your lower back.

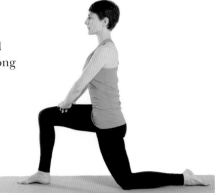

- Start in Four-point Kneeling (*see* p. 77), then bring your right foot forwards. Place your hands on your right thigh and lengthen yourself upright. Keeping a strong connection to your centre, release your weight slightly forwards to open up into the hip flexor.

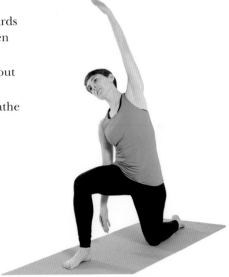

- Breathing in, float the left arm up towards the ceiling, maintaining a space between the arm and the ear.
- Staying strong in your centre, breathe out as you reach the arm over to the right.
- Feel a stretch in the waist and hip. Breathe in to the stretch.

- Release back to centre. Repeat on the other side.

Chapter 2

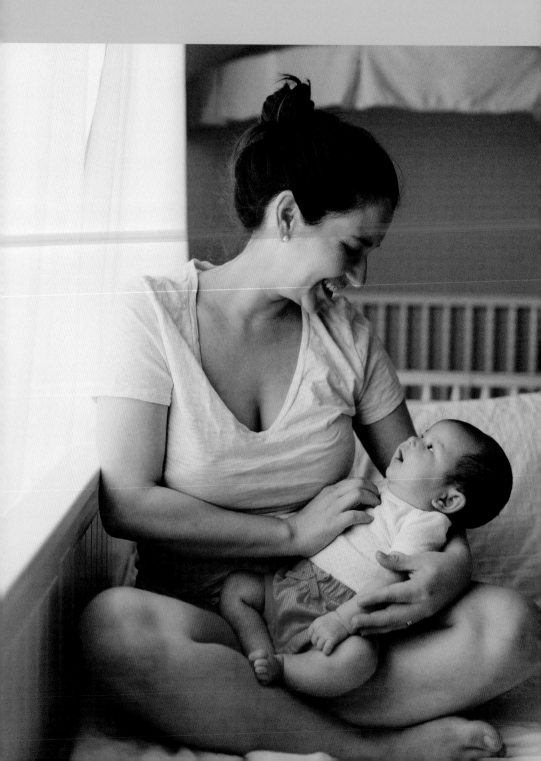

The fourth trimester: birth to three months

The fourth trimester is the immediate postnatal period. Recently, it's become more widely understood that we need to honour this period in a conscious and nurturing way, for our long-term physical recovery as well as our mental and emotional health. The first three months of motherhood is a time of huge transition and change. Bliss, upheaval and mayhem. It will take this whole time, at least, for your emotions and body to settle into a sense of vaguely confident 'normality'. It's totally to be expected that you'll feel discombobulated and chaotic at times. Think of it as starting a new job: you'd imagine that the first few months would be a steep learning curve and that you'd feel way out of your comfort zone. It's no different for your new job as a mother/mum of two/three (or more!). This chapter walks you through the particular demands of this time of your postnatal life and introduces some exercises that are perfect for balancing body and mind at this stage.

In the first few days and weeks after giving birth you'll probably feel bruised and sore, whatever birth experience you've had. Some women feel like a superhero, with such a sense of euphoria that anything seems possible – it can be hard to imagine that you have to take it easy and rest while you're riding this high. But equally, you may fall into the camp of women who feel depleted and exhausted by birth and early days. That was certainly me first time round, and if this is you, please don't push yourself to hold up a façade of 'normal'. Lie down as much as you can. Cuddle your tiny newborn to get the oxytocin flowing and soothe both of your nervous systems; your breathing helps to regulate your baby's breathing. Snuggle with lots of calming skin-to-skin contact in those early days. Eat warming, healing broth. It takes time to complete your metamorphosis into motherhood, and 'normal' takes on a different appearance from now on.

Your emotional health

The newborn phase is a rollercoaster time. It's a watershed of all of the anticipation of the past nearly year, finally holding your baby in your arms (and even more if you've been trying for a while). You will probably feel exhilarated and ecstatic. But you also might feel a bit shocked, indifferent and exhausted – and this is normal, too. Be wary of allowing hundreds of visitors in to see and hold your baby if you really don't feel up to it – and certainly don't be the one making tea if you do. Follow the advice of many a fourth-trimester guru: a week in bed, a week around the bed. It's perfectly acceptable and desirable to enjoy lying down, skin to skin with your baby and not moving very much or expending any energy. Talking to lots of people, 'showing face' and smiling while other people cuddle your new baby is expending energy, both for you and your baby. It is a joyful time taking your baby home, but it is also unprecedentedly stressful, and if you're trying to establish breastfeeding it can have a detrimental effect to have lots of visitors vying for your baby's cuddles or watching you while you're trying to get to grips with a challenging new skill.

Give yourself a break if you don't feel 100 per cent happy every moment. Emotions run high and 'baby blues' are to be expected a few days after birth, usually coinciding with your milk fully coming in (whether you breastfeed or not), the hormonal watershed after having birthed the placenta (your hormone-creating factory for the past nine months) and the exhaustion of 24-hour days taking its toll. If you are feeling very on edge, anxious or detached and depressed by the time your six-week check comes around, please reach out to your health visitor or GP and ask what support there is available. There should be no stigma to mental health issues, so please don't succumb to 'I'm fine' syndrome if you're anything but. Keep a close eye on your mental health for the first year of your baby's life – and beyond. Each phase of motherhood brings different challenges, things get easier but something else always gets harder. Your sleep deprivation might accumulate and have an effect on your resilience. Be kind to yourself. Always come back to your breathing and your awareness of the physical symptoms of stress and anxiety.

Your amazing postnatal body

The immediate postnatal period often feels like your body isn't your own, your baby may have vacated the premises but even if you're not breastfeeding, your boobs will have been taken over by post-birth milk creation. You will rarely have any time when you're not physically connected to your new housemate. And this is amazing in so many beautiful ways, but can occasionally feel like you've lost yourself a bit and you need space without anyone 'on' you. You might have loved your baby bump, and now your belly wobbles like a deflating water balloon and you feel, literally, empty. Internally, it feels like everything's been swapped around, as if all the furniture in your house has been surreptitiously rearranged, and maybe a supporting wall has been knocked down. Now is the

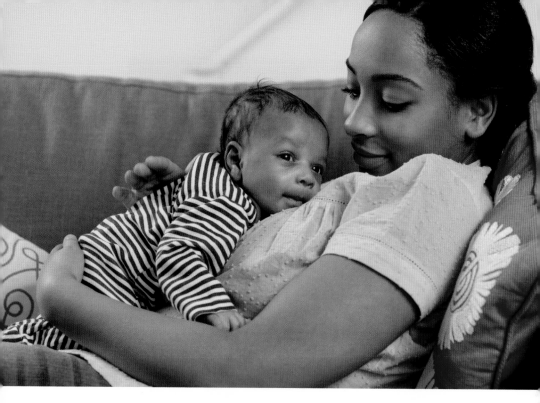

time to focus on reconnecting to your body, re-establishing your breathing, your pelvic floor, your awesome abdominals.

You might even feel despair about your postnatal body, which can trigger deeply held issues with negative body image. It's important to remember that you are vulnerable in body–mind right now, and you'll reap better long-term rewards if you don't rush it. As we discussed previously, it takes time to recover your strength. HIIT, 'body shreds' and Boot Camps are not the way forwards initially, which can be a bitter pill to swallow if you were a gym bunny pre-children. Be patient with yourself. *It's now: it's not forever.* It's really important to take the time to recover fully from childbirth, to help prevent problems with future pregnancies and in your pelvic floor *for life.*

Your six-week check

The six-week GP check – where you are pronounced 'back to normal'. In some surgeries this isn't even viewed as a necessary check any more and you have to request it. If this is the case for your local surgery, please don't skip it, it's really important to check in on your physical recovery and access a forum for asking questions about your healing. This check is not, and never has been, meant to be a 'clearance for exercise', yet for some reason that's what it's understood as being. It generally covers a discussion

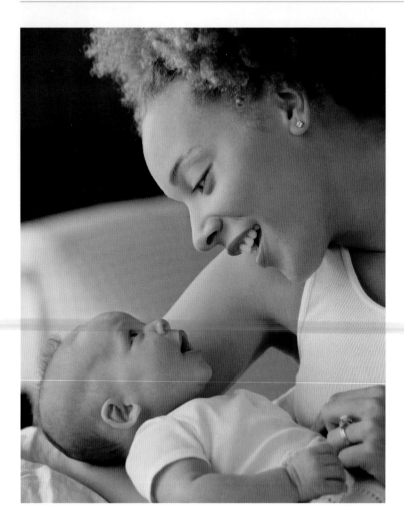

about contraception (although you may feel like this has never felt less relevant) and your mental health in this early period. It rarely comprehensively checks your physical healing. Only a full physio check at this point would truly 'clear you for exercise'. Please speak up if you don't feel that you are being given more than a cursory glance-over. Make sure you ask your GP about:

- *Pelvic floor* – ask to be checked internally if that feels appropriate and safe for you. Ask for *specific* guidance about pelvic floor exercise and describe the pain/discomfort you're experiencing if you're worried. Don't suggest that everything is fine if it's not. Now's the time to speak up. If you ask to be referred to a women's health physio now, it may be that due to waiting lists you wouldn't get an appointment for a few weeks/months anyway, so bear this in mind if the doctor suggests it's 'too soon' to see a physio and tells you to come back in a few weeks. *Ask to be referred now*. It's too easy to postpone this and just hope things will get better in time. Tending to your new baby, it can feel like this actually isn't that important, but it is. *You are important too.* Pelvic floor issues don't magically get better on their own.

- **Diastasis recti** – *ask to have your abdominals* checked. In my experience, it may not be mentioned unless you bring it up, and even then your GP may look nonplussed. If your GP dismisses you, or doesn't seem to know what you're asking, don't be deterred. Don't allow anyone to suggest that this is 'just' a mum issue that is 'normal' and you have to put up with. Ask to be referred to a women's health physio, or get yourself independently to one, or to a postnatal-qualified Pilates trainer so they can check you. *Do not be fobbed off.* This is so important and sadly not something that GPs yet have enough awareness of or time to promote robustly.

It takes six weeks just for your uterus to settle and the blood supply to regulate back to pre-birth levels. Your body will only just have started to assemble itself into its pre-baby organisation at a cellular level. Your connective tissue needs to reconnect. It can take months and months for your hormones to balance to pre-pregnancy levels. If you've had a Caesarean or a birth with intervention, there will be multiple layers of invisible tissue healing going on, which require lengthy rehabilitation *and ample rest.* Giving birth is a huge event. Don't belittle it by assuming that after six weeks you are 'back to normal'.

Birth trauma

If you experienced a traumatic birth and you've been left feeling shaky, panicky and anxious, crying a lot or experiencing flashbacks, don't ignore these feelings as they may be a sign of birth trauma or Post-traumatic Stress Disorder (PTSD), which is increasingly recognised as a condition related to birth. You can request a Birth Debrief: an opportunity to go through your birthing notes with a consultant midwife, at a time that feels right for you. This should be offered as a matter of course by your hospital, particularly if you've had an emergency Caesarean or other surgery, but if not, request it. If your baby is particularly fretful and hard to settle for prolonged periods, remember they have also been through a very traumatic physical event. It might be worth visiting a cranial osteopath who can release and soothe any physical discomfort that your baby might be experiencing post birth. My first (very colicky and distressed) baby benefited hugely from cranial osteopathy, so it's worth trying. Details in the Resources.

What's going on in my body in the fourth trimester?

Your uterus contracts back to its original size in the days after giving birth, which is painful – similar to early labour contractions. This is stimulated particularly by breastfeeding, and it's more intense if it's not your first baby. Establishing breastfeeding is hard, mentally and physically, and is painful initially even if your baby takes to it easily, despite what your health visitor might suggest. You're also very hormonal, so you'll be feeling tender and emotional.

Breathing techniques are so valuable for getting you through these intense early days. If it's your second or subsequent baby, you might be less hit by the enormity of the physical challenge, but you have the added emotional challenge of introducing your new baby into your household of other children and changing the status quo, possibly dealing with demands from your firstborn to 'give the baby back now, we're not keeping him' (true story). All of this brings with it lots of joy but also it's very normal to feel overwhelmed with all the upheaval. So, revisit deep breathing exercises to soothe your nervous system, *every day*.

Pelvic floor awareness exercises are suitable from 24 hours after your birth, whenever you feel ready. Breathing exercises are particularly useful for the first days and weeks after you've had your baby, to relax and soothe your body and soul and to stimulate your circulation and therefore your healing: Legs Up the Wall (*see* p. 114) and Pelvic Floor: Pubic Bone Breathing (*see* p. 102) are especially beneficial. The exercises in this chapter can safely be performed as soon as you feel comfortable – please check with your GP if you have any concerns. Please also wait until 8–12 weeks after Caesarean or vaginal birth with surgical intervention. Gentle, supported rotation and stability exercises such as Chalk Circles (*see* p. 85) and Side-lying Ball Roll (*see* p. 112) can be performed in the initial six-week period *as long as you feel well enough.*

Injuries to the perineum

Birth injuries are no party. You may be told that what you've experienced is 'just a graze', but promise me that you'll speak up if you're still in pain months (or even years) later. Scar tissue build-up can affect how tears heal, impact on your pelvic floor function, and can mean that sex is painful. Women tend to feel shy and nervous about coming forward with these issues. Apparently the *average* time a woman takes to go to her GP with pelvic floor issues is seven years. *Seven years.* Don't suffer in silence.

Tearing, and episiotomy care and recovery

The degrees of tearing are:
- *First degree* – This involves the skin of the perineum and the back of the vagina. These tears are often so small they don't need stitching; in fact they heal better naturally.

- *Second degree* – The skin and back of the vagina, plus the muscles of the perineum are torn. It needs to be stitched, usually by the midwife.
- *Third degree* – This involves the skin, back of the vagina, muscles of the perineum and extends partially or completely through the anal sphincter. Stitches are needed to close these tears, usually performed by a surgeon rather than the midwife.
- *Fourth degree* – This is the same as the third-degree tear, but extends into the rectum. Surgery is needed.

Perineal injuries, grazes or 'tearing', can occur for a number of reasons:
- A rapid or a long, delivery
- Natural perineal stretching being impeded for some reason: pushing too intensely without the expulsive reflex, for example.
- An episiotomy is performed.

It can take up to a month for tears to heal and for stitches to dissolve (small tears with no stitches usually heal faster). In that time you'll probably be in some pain, so make sure you take painkillers if you need to, and breathe deeply. Having an episiotomy or suffering a tear carries the risk of scarring, so at a time that feels right for you, when the area is no longer tender, internal self-massage is a way of stimulating the healing process and breaking down the scar tissue, making sure there is minimal effect on your pelvic floor sensation in the long term.

Bathing in warm water and/or using a cushion can help (a special inflatable cushion can make sitting down more comfortable, or roll up two towels and place them under your thighs, which will take the pressure off the perineum).

If you're still uncomfortable after a few weeks, make sure you speak to your midwife, health visitor or GP.

Here are some tips for this early healing period:
- Keep the cut/tear and surrounding area clean – just use water, no soap products.
- After going to the toilet, pour a jug of warm water over your perineum to rinse it.
- Going for a wee can be painful: it might help if you pee in the bath (just before getting out), or in a warm shower. Take a cup of warm water with you to the toilet and flush over the area straight afterwards to prevent the sting.
- You might be scared to poo because you're worried about pressure on the stitches. This fear causes a lot of extra discomfort and emotional distress. You can ask your midwife, GP or health visitor about medication to help you poo more easily, but deep

breathing should be employed first and foremost. One tip for alleviating pressure on the pelvic floor and avoiding straining is to create a 'squatty potty' by lifting your feet up when sitting on the loo – a toddler step is ideal so even if this is your first baby invest in one now (as you will need it later anyway). Elevating the feet changes the angle of the pelvis, which alters the pressure down into your pelvic floor and can make all the difference when pooing to avoid straining, which can really help prevent or exacerbate prolapse (*see* p. 42).

- After having a poo, make sure you carefully wipe front to back, away from your vagina, to keep the stitches clean.
- Wrap an ice pack or ice cubes in a towel or cloth soaked in diluted tea tree/lavender/witch hazel oil and place on to the affected area, to relieve the pain. You could also soak a sanitary towel with this diluted solution and keep it in the freezer, then place it in your knickers. Or you can now buy ready-made sprays that contain soothing and healing ingredients, such as Spritz for Bitz – which can also be used for Caesarean wound healing (and for your baby's nappy rash).
- Restart pelvic floor *awareness* exercises as soon as you can after birth. They enhance blood circulation and aid the healing process.

Healing your pelvic floor

Although you might not think it's appropriate if you're sore and tired, pelvic floor awareness 'exercises' can and should start around 24 hours after birth, even if you had a Caesarean birth. If you've had stitches, don't be scared about disturbing them – actually the opposite is true. Trauma to the pelvic floor can begin to heal if you encourage blood circulation to the area, which will help to reduce swelling. All of the pelvic floor exercises included are appropriate here.

As your healing progresses and you become more mobile, start to exercise your pelvic floor in different positions: lying down, sitting, standing. Think about your pelvic floor and connecting to your centre in your regular daily activities, which is when you most need them: when you're standing up from sitting, picking your baby up, pushing your baby's buggy, carrying shopping while putting your baby in the car seat, etc.

We need to start viewing birth injury as just that, *injury*. Injured muscle doesn't reactivate without conscious attention and rehab. A professional footballer wouldn't go back onto the pitch having torn her hamstring before having extensive physio to heal properly. We need to view a torn pelvic floor with the same mentality.

> ## Tip
>
> For Caesarean post-birth care tips – see the next chapter. If you had a vaginal birth with surgical intervention, a lot of the Caesarean chapter applies to you as well. Surgery, even if not under emotionally traumatic circumstances, is *trauma* for your body, and there are implications for the length of your healing when incisions and stitches are involved.

SNIFF, FLOP, DROP
Stage 1

This is a technique created by the pelvic physiotherapist Maeve Whelan, whose details you can find in the Resources, as a way of developing your ability to *relax* your pelvic floor.

1. *Start in Relaxation Position* (*see* p. 56), or you can also do this sitting down – or standing. Play around with pelvic floor awareness exercises in all positions, ultimately.

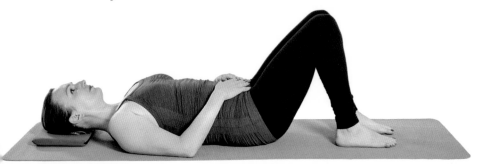

2. *SNIFF: inhale through the nose*
- Breathe in through the nose, allow the stomach to FLOP, keeping it soft.
- Stay on the in-breath for three seconds, keeping the stomach soft. Practise this for a few breaths.
- Allow your in-breath to be longer than your out-breath. Your out-breath should almost disappear: this means you've let all your tension go.
- Your out-breath should sound like a dynamic sigh: 'hah', as if you're cleaning your glasses.
- The less effort, the better the connection will be.

3. *FLOP: fill out your stomach softly*
- Allow your stomach to soften into your fingertips placed under your ribs on your upper abdomen.

4. *DROP: release or open at the back passage – backwards*
- When your abdomen is soft and filling out as the diaphragm descends, you can then expect to feel a connection to the pelvic floor as it too lets go – the DROP.

THE LESS EFFORT, THE BETTER – imagine going into a state of complete relaxation and almost meditation.

PELVIC ELEVATOR
Stage 1

Imagine that your pelvic floor is a lift in a building. We have ground floor (your pelvic floor at rest), levels one, two and three. There is also a basement floor below ground floor.

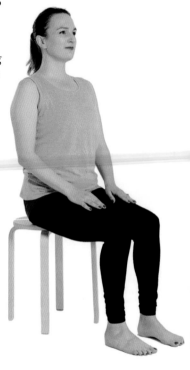

- Sit on a chair, feet hip-width apart. You could also do this while lying in Relaxation Position (*see* p. 56).
- Breathe in, wide into your sides.
- Breathe out, connect to your centre, visualise closing the lift doors. Imagine the sit bones drawing towards each other (without clenching your buttocks).
- Breathe in, maintain that engagement.
- Breathe out as the lift travels to the first floor.
- Breathe in to pause this engagement.
- Breathe out and take the lift to the second floor.
- Breathe in, pause.
- Breathe out and take the lift up to the top floor, as far as you can without bracing.
- Soften your shoulders and jaw as you hold the connection.
- Breathe in as you descend to the next floor slowly, then lower to the next.
- When you reach the ground floor, soften your muscles fully to lower to the basement floor. 'Open the doors' of the lift and release your pelvic floor muscles completely.
- Repeat up to 5 times.

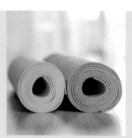

CASE STUDY

Julie, mum of three

Postnatally, I found it hard to find my pelvic floor again, never mind strengthen it. Pilates really helped that.

PELVIC FLOOR: LIFT AND PULSE
Stage 1

The pelvic floor has to be strong for endurance. But it also has to have the power for short bursts of strength. This exercise develops the 'fast-twitch' muscle fibres, which are responsible for those shorter bursts of movement and energy. For example, chicken wings contain lots of fast-twitch fibres, enabling the chicken to take flight if they get scared – fast-twitch fibres are quick to respond, but also fatigue after a short burst of energy.

The pelvic floor needs both stamina and speed: it needs the fast-twitch capability for rapid response when you cough, laugh, sneeze or jump around, as well as needing stamina and marathon endurance when your baby is making her descent out into the world. In the postnatal period, stress incontinence is a common issue. If your rapid response team isn't mobilised soon enough, sneezing or coughing can lead to embarrassing leaks. This exercise is a good training drill to prepare your pelvic floor team for those 'emergencies' that require strength without a moment to lose!

Once you've got it, practise this in a number of different positions: standing, sitting, lying. This will help create the muscle memory (and the habit) for it to be more effective in your daily life.

- Breathe normally. After an out-breath, fully engage your pelvic floor.
- Hold for about five seconds, in the space between breaths.

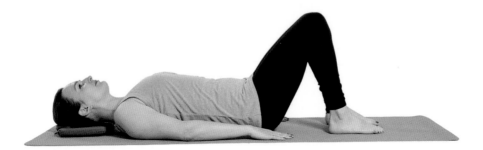

- Release and breathe in deeply into your belly, imagining your diaphragm taking up space within your centre.
- Repeat and this time lift and pulse 5 times.
- Release completely, breathing in.
- Repeat around 6 times, building up to 10 pulses if you can.
- Remember 10, 10, 3: We won't pee with 10, 10, 3 (*see* p. 61)

PELVIC FLOOR: PUBIC BONE BREATHING
Stage 1

We're conditioned to hold our bellies in – we suck our tummies in tight and hold our breath, 'to look better'. Holding your tummy leads to a lot of pressure within the abdomen – intra-abdominal pressure – temporarily squishing your internal organs and increasing the load on your pelvic floor, rather than creating any useful strength or muscle balance.

This exercise allows you to connect to your belly through your breath, release your diaphragm fully and relax all of the muscles around your abdomen and your pelvic floor. You may have noticed that newborns naturally breathe this way: when a baby takes in a breath its belly inflates hugely like a balloon, then releases back with its in-breath. We need to learn from the newborn's pure instinctive breath.

- Start lying on your back, head on a small cushion, knees bent, arms relaxed with hands on the belly, fingertips resting towards your pubic bone. Release your weight into the floor. Feel the heaviness of your head, ribcage, pelvis.

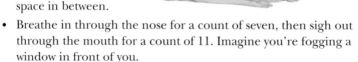

- Bring your awareness to your breath. Notice the in-breath, the out-breath, the space in between.

- Breathe in through the nose for a count of seven, then sigh out through the mouth for a count of 11. Imagine you're fogging a window in front of you.

- Bring your awareness to your tummy and pelvis, the sensation of your fingertips on your pubic bone.

- Breathe in and imagine sending your breath towards your pubic bone, down through the torso, the ribcage opens and the belly inflates with the breath.

- As you breathe out, notice the fall in your abdomen as the breath recedes.

- See whether you can channel your breath deep down towards the belly and pelvis, imagine it like a soft wave travelling down the body and washing away any tension.

- On the out-breath, feel your tummy soften and imagine the pelvis wide and open, and completely relaxed.

- Practise releasing the jaw by changing the sounds of your out-breath. Experiment with a 'haaaaaah' sound, a long audible sigh.

TABLE TOP LEG EXTEND

Stage 1

This is to challenge the deep activation of your abdominals and work into the hip muscles. We need to keep the pelvis stable while the legs move.

- Start in Four-point Kneeling (*see* p. 77).

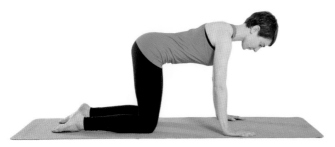

- Breathe in to lengthen and prepare. As you breathe out, slide your right leg out behind you, keeping the foot in contact with the ground.

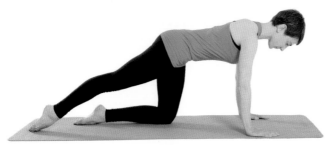

- Breathe in to return. Repeat on that side, up to 10 times.
- Repeat on the other leg.
- Rest back into Rest Position (*see* p. 81).

Watchpoints

Imagine you have a mirror in front of you on the mat to check if you're 'swinging' your torso or hips to the side of your sliding leg. If you are, or if your hips have to 'shift' to bring the knee back underneath you, *you're not working your deep core*. Try to maintain stability with the torso centred.

If you're recruiting your muscles correctly, the leg will glide in and out with no visible effect on the torso. Think *length* from head to tail, long waist on each side.

THIGH STIRS
Stage 1

This exercise can be performed with a band, or without (which requires a bit more control). It improves the circulation in your lower body, in the pelvis and your legs.

- Start in Relaxation Position (*see* p. 56). Float one knee in towards you (Single Knee Folds, *see* p. 71) and place a stretchy band around the back of your thigh. Hold the ends of the band in one hand and release your elbows to the floor.

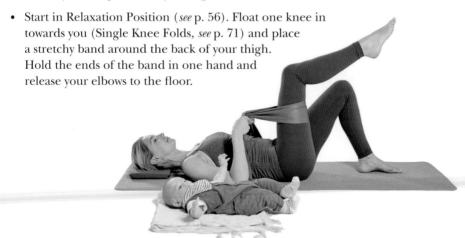

- Circle the thighbone clockwise, slowly. Imagine stirring the leg in its socket like a cocktail stick in a glass. Keep the movement in the thighbone and not leading with the knee or the foot. Try to maintain heaviness in the pelvis, moving the thighbone without rotating in the spine or moving the bottom on the floor.
- Repeat the circle 5 or 6 times and then reverse.

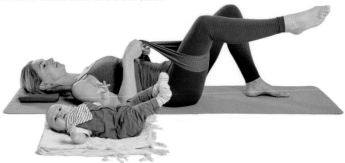

- You can also create infinity circles, figures-of-eight, to really oil the hip joint.
- Repeat on the other leg.

Watchpoint
Check in with your alignment: shoulders heavy, waist long, pelvis relaxed and grounded.

WINDSCREEN WIPER LEGS
Stage 1

This is great for encouraging circulation to the hip and pelvic area, which can be prone to stiffness in the early postnatal period.

- Lie in Relaxation Position (*see* p. 56), feet slightly wider than hip-width apart.
- Breathe in to lengthen and prepare.
- As you breathe out, send the thighs to the left with control, allowing them to separate and move independently from each other. Breathe in to the hip joints and allow the stretch to open there.

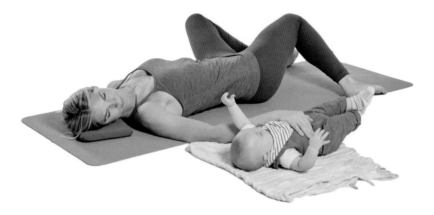

- Breathe out to move to the other side. The hip movement will travel into a rotation of the pelvis and lumbar spine.
- Enjoy the stretch of the waist and hip, while keeping the shoulders heavy and open.

EXERCISE AND BREASTFEEDING

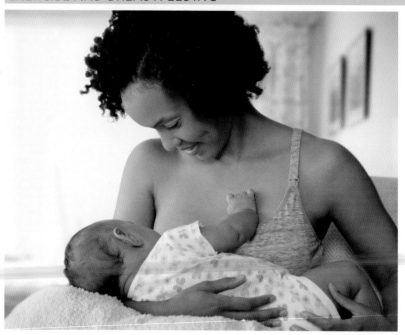

Rest is incredibly important for milk production, so particularly if you've had a challenging birth experience, prioritise lots of time for simply breathing and lying down. This is not wasted time, it's so valuable and necessary. Imagine trying to use your phone when the battery has run out – and then see yourself as requiring recharging in exactly the same way. Once you're ready, there is no research to suggest that *gentle* exercise has a negative effect on your breastmilk supply. However, it's often devilishly uncomfortable to lie on your front with the two tender, rock-hard milk-making orbs on your front, which means that you may not feel comfortable performing exercises on your front, or even some Four-point Kneeling exercises. Take care, don't lie on your front if your boobs are sore, and only do as many repetitions as feel comfortable for you – and don't tire yourself out. Make sure you drink enough water – breastfeeding is thirsty work – so have a glass of water at least every time you feed.

It's a good idea to feed baby before you do any Pilates. If your boobs are full, chances are they'll feel uncomfortable, and any amount of movement may stimulate your milk, so it's advisable to wear breast pads to avoid too much leakage. Although to be honest, you'll be so used to leaking after a while that you won't really mind.

You might want to keep the range of movement of some arm exercises smaller and controlled. Anything that involves reaching your arms over your head or stretching away from the body, such as with Chalk Circles or Shoulder Stretch (*see* p. 85 and 66), might cause tenderness early on.

POSTURE CHECK FOR FEEDING
Stage 1

Forward leaning when feeding your baby constantly can literally become a pain in the neck. In some ways, aches and pains are inevitable as a new mum, but being mindful of your posture will go some way to avoiding the worst of it, and more importantly, ensure that you're not entrenching pain into your body for the long term.

When you're feeding, particularly when breastfeeding but this is also relevant if you're bottle feeding, bring your baby up to you rather than hunching forwards for your boob to reach your baby's mouth. Prop baby or your elbow up with enough pillows and cushions, to support his body closer to your own without strain. Always remember to bring baby to boob, rather than lowering your boob to baby.

Notice what kind of position you adopt when you're feeding. Often, we're crouched and distorted, balancing on our toes with a crick neck, to ensure that our baby is happy and comfortable – mother yourself a bit. Bolster your back and arm with pillows, make sure you have a footrest if you need it, and stretch out your body afterwards, even just very briefly, by doing a Shoulder Stretch (*see* p. 66) and the following Neck Stretch. You'll avoid longer-term neck, lower back and foot issues by taking a moment to consider your own comfort.

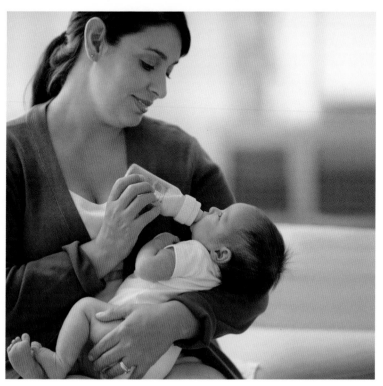

NECK STRETCH AND RELEASE
Stage 1

After each feed, try to make sure you do this gentle stretch.

- Take a long, deep breath in and sigh the breath out through your lips, as if you're fogging a window in front of you. Relax your jaw and soften your face.
- Sitting upright, nod your left ear down to your left shoulder, looking forwards.
- Raise your hand to the side of your head and place a gentle pressure to increase the stretch. Return slowly to centre, then repeat to the right.

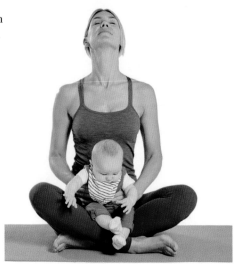

- Return slowly to centre, then look up, opening the throat.

- Slowly look down, nodding your chin to your chest.

STRETCH AND RELAXATION SEQUENCE

The next few exercises are perfect for relaxing and releasing tension at the end (or middle!) of a mothering day. Pick just one for a micro meditation moment, or, do all five together and it should only take 10 minutes of your evening (feel free to linger for longer).

HIP FLEXOR STRETCH
Stage 1

- Start in Relaxation Position (*see* p. 56).
- Float one leg in towards your chest.
- Take your hands around the front of your knee and draw that knee deeper in towards your body.

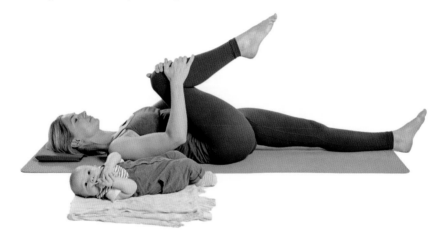

- At the same time, lengthen the other leg away along the floor. Feel the front of the hip open and release.
- Allow the tailbone and the shoulders to soften into the floor.

HIP FLEXOR STRETCH WITH ROTATION AND HALF SNOW ANGELS
Stage 1

- From Hip Flexor Stretch (*see* p. 109), drop your foot into the thigh of the resting leg.
- With the opposite arm, take hold of your knee and guide it across towards the floor, twisting the hips. Extend your other arm out along the floor at shoulder height and look towards the palm of your hand.

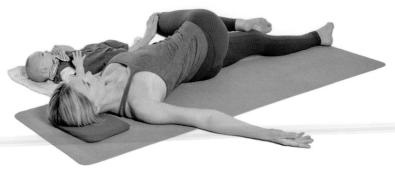

- As you breathe into the rotation and gently stretch into your spine and hips, travel the resting arm up above your head, maintaining contact with the floor. Then, reach the arm out and down to the hip, as if drawing a snow angel. Repeat 3 or 4 times as you breathe deeply.

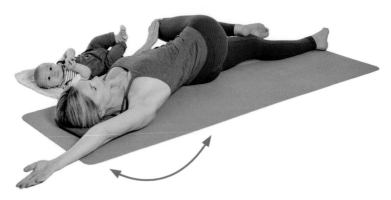

- Repeat on the other side.

GLUTE STRETCH
Stage 1

- From Relaxation Position (*see* p. 56), fold your right knee in towards your chest.
- Fold the right ankle on top of the left knee.
- Carefully, with control, float the left knee in towards you and hold on behind the thigh. Feel the stretch in the right side of your bottom.

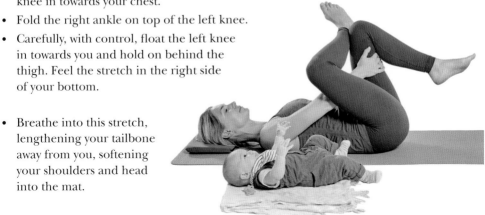

- Breathe into this stretch, lengthening your tailbone away from you, softening your shoulders and head into the mat.

- Stay here, deepening into your stretch for a few breaths.

ADDUCTOR STRETCH
Stage 1

This is such a therapeutic position to be in postnatally. If you do nothing else, take a moment out of your day to lie on your back, breathing long and deeply, allowing the back of your body to release and open, and letting go of any tension you are holding on to around your shoulders, pelvis and inner thighs. Take care if you've had PGP and avoid if any pelvic pain lingers.

- From Relaxation Position (*see* p. 56), fold one knee followed by the other in to your chest.
- Connect the insides of the feet and reach your arms through the centre of your thighs to hold on to your shin/ankles.
- Allow your inner thighs to release.
- Breathe long and deep.

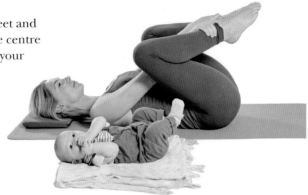

SIDE-LYING BALL ROLL
Stage 1

This exercise massages the muscles between your shoulder blades, releasing stiffness and tension. It stimulates the natural pelvic floor response and gently reawakens natural movement in the upper back.

- Lie on your side, with your bottom arm lengthened underneath your head and knees bent, feet in line with your bottom. Place your top arm outstretched in front of you, at shoulder height. Rest your palm on top of a small ball.
- Breathe in to lengthen the spine and connect to your centre.

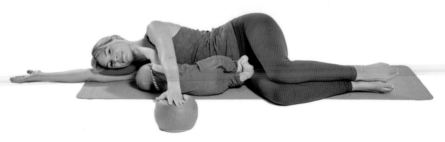

- Breathe out as you roll the ball forwards and away from you, allowing your ribcage to roll forwards to follow your arm. Keep your pelvis upright.

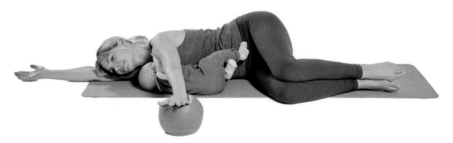

- Breathe in and roll the ball back towards you, moving from the shoulder blade without bending the arm or wrist.
- Repeat up to 10 times.

Watchpoint

Keep the arm straight as you draw the ball back in towards you. It should be a movement of the shoulder blade on the ribcage, not in the elbow and wrist.

SEATED PELVIC ROLL-BACK
Stage 1

This is a gentle way of activating your deep pelvic floor and abdominal muscles. It's perfect for an easy way of tuning into your pelvic floor and healing diastasis recti, as you may be sitting on the floor a lot with your baby at this time. It's also great if you're spending a lot of time feeding: you can adapt it for sitting on the sofa, to be aware of your sitting posture and wake up your spine.

- Sitting tall on your sit bones, lengthen your legs out in front of you at hip-width apart, then bend your knees to take your feet flat on the floor. Breathe in to lengthen into the spine, and take your hands behind your thighs.

- Breathe out, and feel the pelvic floor lift. Place some pressure into your hands as you tuck your tailbone underneath you and curl your spine into a C-curve, evenly rolling through each bone and curling your chin towards your chest lightly – imagine soft length in your neck.

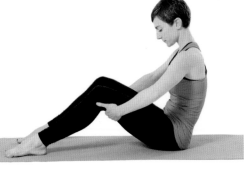

- *If you feel strong enough* and can do this without abdominal doming, from here lengthen this C-shape back, lowering your hands slightly and deepening your connection with the lower abdominals to support your weight. The energy should be coming from your pelvic floor and deep abdominals, not from your hips gripping. Breathe in to lengthen into this position.

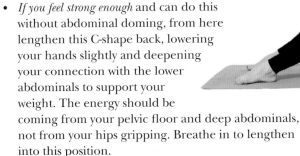

- Breathe out to return the C-shape above the hips.
- Breathe in to lengthen back into neutral, fully releasing your pelvic floor engagement, then open your heart centre to extend into the upper spine. Keep the neck long, without too much extension into the neck.
- Return to neutral, and repeat the whole sequence up to 5 times.

LEGS UP THE WALL
Stage 1

This is a restorative position, a place to practise some deep breathing and release the tension of the day, from your muscles and your mind.

- Bring your mat towards the wall. Sit facing to the side, with your hips close to the wall. Rotate your legs towards the wall as you descend on to the mat. Ease yourself down on to your side, then roll on to your back. Have a pillow/s underneath your head and torso if you need to. Float your legs in and rest them against the wall, softly bent. Place your hands on your tummy, or on the floor.

- Breathe in and feel your hand on your tummy rise. Notice any sensations.

- Breathe out and feel your tummy lower and soften.

- Allow your legs to feel heavy and totally relaxed.

- Stay in this position for as long as feels comfortable for you.

Tip

You can take 'legs over the sofa' instead if your hamstrings are particularly tight: lie on your floor and drape your legs over the sofa, knees bent.

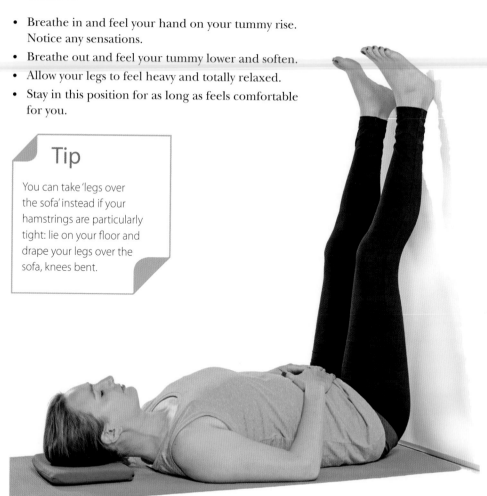

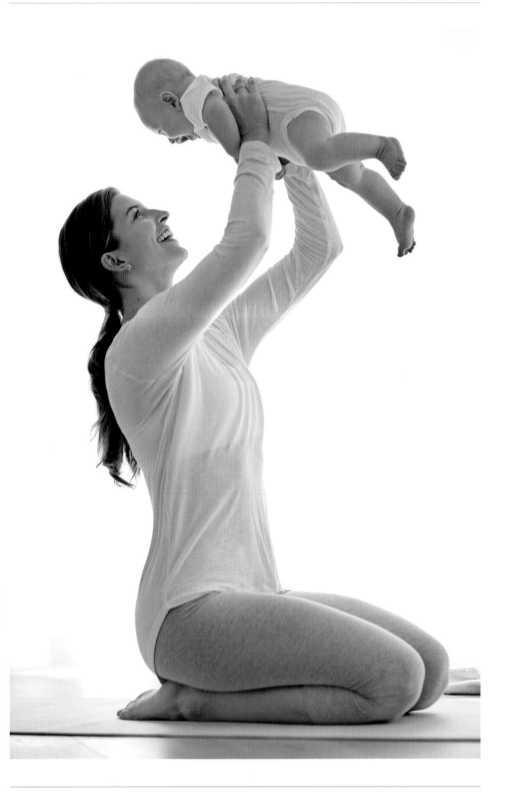

WORKOUTS FOR THE FOURTH TRIMESTER

These routines are perfect for doing with your baby next to you or underneath you in Four-point Kneeling (*see* p. 77). You are able to have eye contact throughout each movement and press down to give your baby a kiss, while continuing to focus on your movement and breath. Remember that you are enabling their development by having them by your side so please don't feel guilty about exercising with them: this is 5-star entertainment for them! Gazing at mama is deeply stimulating for your baby. What's more, simply by moving with them you enhance their muscular development, coordination and motor skills, and deepen your attachment and bond.

5-minute workout	
Relaxation: Pelvic Floor: Pubic Bone Breathing 102	
Pelvic Tilts 57	
Hip Rolls 87	
Hip Flexor Stretch 109	
Centring in Four-point Kneeling 77	

10-minute workout	
Relaxation Position 56	
Sniff, Flop, Drop 99	
Pelvic Floor: Lift and Pulse 101	
Compass 75–6	
Knee Drops 69	
Hip Rolls 87	
Ribcage Closure 74	
Cat–Cow 80	

WORKOUTS FOR THE FOURTH TRIMESTER

20-minute workout	
Scarf Breathing 58	
Roll-downs Against the Wall 79	
Wall Posture Check and Side Reach 64	
Shoulder Stretch 66	
Relaxation Position: Pelvic Floor Lift and Pulse 101	
Spine Curls 82	

20-minute workout cont.	
Band Pull with Knee Drop 70	
Leg Slides 68	
Windscreen Wiper Legs 105	
Glute Stretch 111	
Cat–Cow 80	
Chalk Circles 85–6	
Legs Up the Wall 114	

Chapter 3

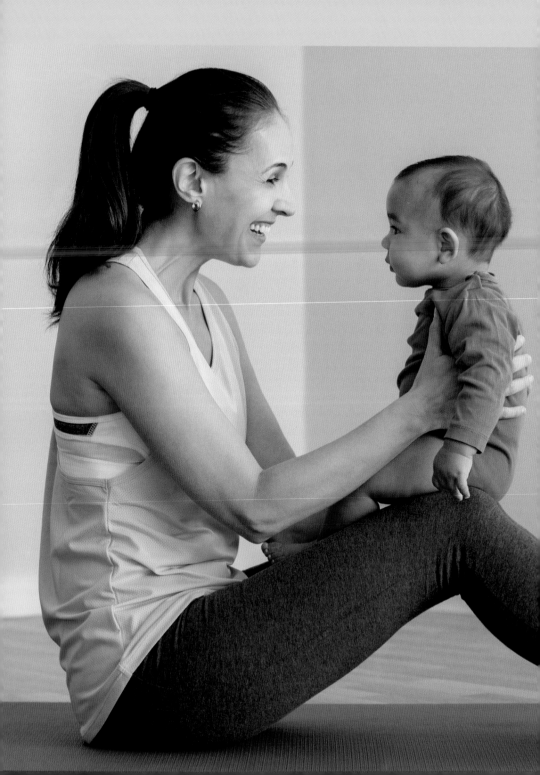

Caesarean recovery

After you've had an abdominal birth, whether planned or not, when you leave hospital you can feel as if you've been let loose with absolutely no guidance about how to help yourself on this crucial road to recovery. It's particularly nerve-wracking if this is your first experience of surgery. Not to mention the 'too posh to push' refrain that implies that abdominal birth is an 'easy' option. Often, we're shaken by how painful and slow post-Caesarean recovery can be. All of the exercises in this chapter are appropriate for your recovery: you may have a bit more work to do at Stage 1, Awareness because your surgery will have severed nerve endings, so you must take time to soften tension, rebuild connections and rewire your circuit.

Top post-surgery tips

o Breathe, and take it slow. Your nervous system needs soothing out of fight-or-flight mode in order to kick-start your physical healing. You *must* rest to enable the healing process.

o Nourish. Your collagen (the main structural protein forming building blocks of your connective tissue) needs proper fuel to heal your injured tissue. Nutrition is so important for the healing process and this is often completely overlooked by new mums. Think chicken soup, lots of broth and healing protein.

o Hydrate. Your connective tissue needs adequate water to renew itself.

Seek advice from a women's health physio. Don't *fear* movement – but equally, don't do too much too soon. It's a tricky balance of just enough but not too much. We need to adopt a kind of 'suck it and see' approach of testing the waters gradually, reviewing how your body reacts each time. This chapter will offer you ways to feel like you're 'getting somewhere' without undermining your long-term recovery.

Begin with your **Stage 1 Awareness** exercises from Chapter 2 as soon as you feel strong and confident enough – that is, literally in the first 24 hours. Then, after about 8–12 weeks, proceed to the **Stage 2 Foundation** exercises. All of the exercises in this book are relevant for you, once you have worked through to reconnect your deep core muscles, but the ones I have selected in this chapter are particularly appropriate for the experience that your body has had with surgery, in the first four to five months post birth (and beyond;

seven years post Caesarean, I still have some numbness and altered sensation in my abdominals).

A quarter of women who give birth now do so abdominally rather than vaginally. It's a very common operation. But – it is *major surgery*. Your recovery must take into account the additional layers of tissue that need to heal compared to a vaginal birth without intervention, even if you 'feel totally fine'. Not to mention the effects of a prolonged labour, and any emotional trauma, if yours was an emergency Caesarean. We use our abdominal muscles for *everything* in life – for breathing, coughing, sneezing, moving, lifting, winding the bobbin up... – abdominal surgery hugely impacts on your daily experience for a while.

Remember there is *no failure* in birth. Abdominal birth is just as legitimate as vaginal birth. Whatever the circumstances of your Caesarean, you may have complex feelings about it. Especially if there has been an element of trauma in your birth story, you'll need to learn how to let go of your judgements of yourself to enable your full recovery. Sometimes emotional healing seems too 'big', too heavy to approach. But, just like any scar tissue, if left alone it becomes packed down into your being, hardens like limescale in a kettle, and begins to affect your wellbeing and vitality.

Focusing on your physical recovery is a good place to start: all of the exercises in this chapter will also ultimately begin to nurture your nervous system and emotional recovery. Both physically and emotionally, this may be an ongoing journey, *and this is OK*. Don't beat yourself up.

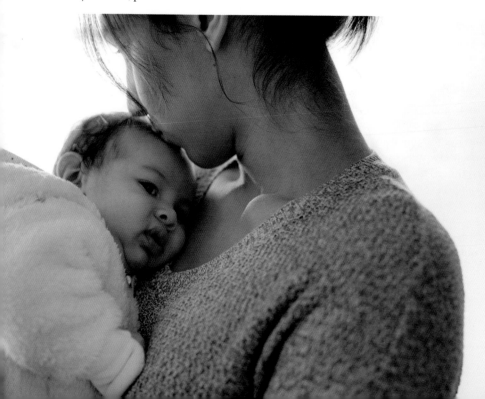

EXPERT ADVICE
How to get out of bed post abdominal surgery

Kate Fry

As a physio, I really emphasise the importance of learning how to get out of bed in the weeks after major abdominal surgery. Always roll to one side and bring the legs around to the edge of the bed, using the arms to push you up. By using this method you put less pressure on the stitches and abdominals. Early mobilisation is important post C-section as it helps reduce respiratory problems, back pain and DVT (deep vein thrombosis). So, as creaky as you may feel, get up and walk slowly around your hospital bed as soon as you can.

Women's health physio, Pilates teacher, and mum of two

When you do get up, stand up tall. You may want to stoop over to protect your belly, and feel like you're going to burst your stitches. Honestly, you won't, and the taller you can stand, the better your chance of allowing your body to realign itself properly.

As a broad guideline, you'll be told not to drive for six weeks, and that your recovery will take 'up to 12 weeks'. This is a huge simplification: for some women it takes a lot longer, others feel totally great after four weeks and can't understand why they might have to take it easy. Each body is different. Even if you 'feel totally fine', treat your body as you would your newborn baby: with compassion and tenderness. Start first with your breathing and posture, then become more aware of your core connection: pelvic floor strengthening and low-level mobility such as pelvic mobility exercises and Spine Curls (*see* p. 82).

Tip

Healing straight after surgery

If you're reading this before you give birth: know that you can enhance your recovery in the first 24 hours post birth. As your anaesthetic is wearing off you can begin to stimulate your circulation. The anaesthetic will mean that you have no feeling in your bottom half, and you won't be able to move your legs. As soon as you begin to feel sensation coming back into your legs, point and flex your feet, circle your ankles. It's not too much effort, and hopefully you'll be calmly having skin-to-skin time with your newborn at this stage.

Pointing and flexing stimulates the calf, getting blood moving around your body again, and is very important to avoid blood clots. It will gently ensure that when you do get up and about – and it's recommended that you start to have a short walk around your bed/ward as soon as you can – you'll be less likely to feel like a complete zombie.

Tip

Why am I told I can't drive and lift things?

So, why can't you drive? Apart from insurance reasons, the act of driving can be quite physical, requiring instant reactions and core strength when e.g. you're reversing/turning corners, and having to be able to brake suddenly if required. All of these use your deep abdominal muscles and require full torso control and mobility in order for them to be performed safely. Sneezing will be painful for the first few weeks, so performing a three-point-turn, for example, would simply be too challenging – which highlights just how much you utilise your core in daily situations. It's just not safe to drive while you're in pain or lacking full mobility, and it's also not advisable to drive while using strong pain medication.

Similarly, lifting utilises your core strongly, increasing the intra-abdominal pressure. So, it will not only potentially be painful to lift heavy items (such as a wriggly toddler or a car seat with a baby in it), but will also be placing a lot of strain on your pelvic floor, your pelvis and back. Stressed tissue won't be able to heal as quickly, and this puts you at risk of wound infection or prolonged pain.

What happens in a Caesarean operation?

A Caesarean section is a common, and safe, operation, but the fact remains – it's major surgery. We rarely have the rehabilitation space (sleep, rest, follow-up care and information, physio) afterwards as we might do for other major surgery, as we have our new and demanding tiny housemate to look after. Understanding a bit more about what actually happens in the surgery may allow you to see why respecting your recovery is so important – and why there is a lot more going on when it comes to healing after a Caesarean than there is for a straightforward vaginal birth.

After the anaesthetic, an incision is made through the abdominal and uterine wall, to create a window to birth your baby through. A classical incision (vertical, underneath the navel down to the pubic bone), is only rarely used in extenuating circumstances, such as in the presence of fibroids or uterine tumours. The lower segment horizontal (or 'bikini line'), incision is most common. Healing and mobility are more easily achieved after this incision, so the outcome is better for maternal recovery and there's less risk of scar rupture in future pregnancies.

The incision has to go through four layers: skin, fat, fascia (connective tissue) and finally into your uterus. Each layer may

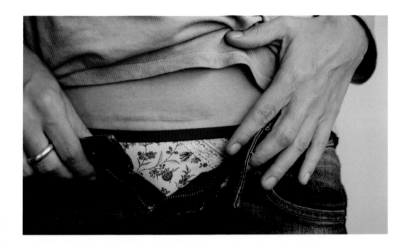

be sutured (stitched) individually – so your final wound 'stitch' is only the visible layer of multiple levels of healing going on. There is no incision made to any muscle except that of the uterus. Your abdominal muscles are instead pulled away from the area to allow access to your baby. The rectus abdominis (six-pack muscle) is pulled apart at its central connective site of the linea alba – which means that, even if you didn't have diastasis recti before your birth then there's more likelihood of compromised strength here after your surgery. You may be sutured with skin clips, dissolving stitches or a subcutaneous skin suture, which is like a thread that runs along the wound site, tying each side together (much easier to remove than individual stitches). Which is used varies from surgeon to surgeon, and depends on various other factors.

Immediate post-Caesarean healing tips

- The first few days/week will be painful. In the immediate aftermath, focus on your breath and gently moving as much as you can to maintain healthy circulation and help your gassy belly release. You'll be tender and bruised. Maybe in heart, soul AND body. So be kind to yourself.
- Wound care: please call your midwife/GP if you're in an inordinate amount of pain, have any fever or if the wound is weeping or is open. I kept a maternity pad in my pants to protect the wound. You can buy Caesarean bands, which do a similar job. It's particularly important to allow a bit of protection if you have older children who might climb on you and inadvertently bash into it. Keep the wound dry by patting it gently after showers/if you're sweating.
- You will have trapped wind – a very common side-effect of abdominal surgery. It may appear (oddly) as very strong

shoulder pain. The pain can be so severe that some mums panic that they're having some kind of heart attack. Peppermint tea can help (although please read up on the possible effects of peppermint tea on breastmilk supply), as can deep breathing and moving your body gently.

- Don't judge yourself. I looked in the mirror and tried to hold in my newly vacant tummy, and nothing happened. It stayed there, stoically still, like a water balloon strapped to my front. This is normal.
- Breathe. Really properly breathe. You need to wake up your belly to its healing journey.
- Drink enough water. Eat enough protein – your tissue and collagen are working their little socks off to heal. Help them by giving them the right fuel.

Abdominal massage

Massage: *the* most crucial piece of advice for Caesarean long-term recovery. I still have pain from scar tissue build-up, which causes pain and stiffness in my hip. It possibly wouldn't be so bad if I'd known about the benefits of massage. Show your tummy some love – this applies after all birth but is particularly appropriate after Caesarean.

A few weeks postnatally – after about eight weeks is ideal – begin to regularly massage your tummy. This not only allows you to foster a bit of self-compassion, and to help to tone and deflate your post-birth tummy with some nourishing body oil (use one that's high in skin-loving Vitamin E, such as rosehip seed oil), but it also has a very important effect of hydrating and moving the tissues, breaking down areas of stuck fibres and helping to prevent adhesions (*see* box, opposite). Massage brings warmth to the scar tissue and the area

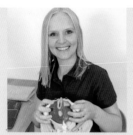

EXPERT ADVICE

Danielle White

Part of your recovery is being able to let go, and connecting to your tummy through massage is an extremely powerful way to do so. As women, we often have little love for our tummy, regularly sucking the muscles in tight, and extra tension after birth can sometimes impact healing. Self-massage helps reconnect to these muscles to help them to let go, allowing you to move your whole body more easily. Not only that, there is strong research to suggest that massage can help improve bowel movements, which in turn helps alleviate pressure on your pelvic floor, scar and diastasis recti.

Women's Health and Wellness Coach, Soft Tissue Therapist, Holistic Core Restore® Coach

around the wound, improves vasodilation (the widening of blood vessels), lymph drainage and blood flow to the area, and may help to prevent adhesions from forming. Plus it's an immensely healing thing to do, to connect to your tummy. Massage as close to your scar site as you comfortably can, and as the months go by and you feel ready (from around 10–12 weeks), massage the scar itself.

I personally, first time round, couldn't bring myself to even look at my scar until 10 weeks after birth, let alone touch it. I didn't breathe deeply, and didn't massage it at all. I only learned about the healing benefits of conscious breathing and massage after having my second baby. A common side-effect of trauma is to entirely block something out so that you don't have to approach it or relive the emotions. If this resonates for you, then at a time that feels safe, try to connect physically to your scar area. Even if this means simply lying and taking your hands on to your lower belly scar site (*see* Pelvic Floor: Pubic Bone Breathing, p. 102), sending your breath and awareness to that space. A lot of emotions may come up, and this is entirely normal. Acknowledging these feelings is the first step to coming to terms with them. However, if it feels very distressing or overwhelming to touch your scar, or it triggers flashbacks about your birth, stop. You may be suffering from birth trauma or post-traumatic stress disorder (PTSD) and you should try to reach out for help and guidance (useful contacts in the Resources).

If I had my first postnatal time again, and if I had known as much about the development of scar tissue as I do now, I would have dedicated time to breathing and *acknowledging* the trauma that

Tip

It's never too late – if you're *years* postnatal and you're reading this, don't worry or berate yourself. You can begin self-massage today and still make a difference to how your lower abdomen looks and feels.

What are adhesions?

Adhesions are bands of fibrous tissue that form when connective tissue sticks together, a bit like Velcro or superglue. Normally, fascia (connective tissue) is well lubricated and glides easily against all neighbouring fascia and organs, but surgery (and this includes ERPC/D&C surgery after miscarriage – evacuation of retained products of conception/dilation and curettage) can mean that fibres become attached to surrounding fibres and form a hard, stuck mass of scar tissue. This can be the invisible cause of much discomfort within the scar/pelvic area post Caesarean in the years after birth, and so it's important to do what you can to try to prevent them forming. It can make your abdomen particularly tender, and cause pain with movement or stretching. The pain might not be felt on the scar site but referred, even in the hip or lower back, which means you might not connect the pain to your surgery.

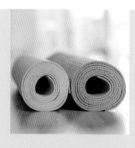

CASE STUDY

Kate, mum of two

After the birth of my son I was a mess, after a 29-hour labour that ended up in an emergency C-section. Five hours later, I was told to get up to look after my baby … but there wasn't anyone there to tell me or help me get up… I wet myself as soon as I stood up (probably the final straw in a long, horrid labour) so I ended up bursting into tears in the middle of the ward! My poor husband nearly started crying when he saw me as well. SUCH a bad day…

my body had been through. I didn't, and partly as a result of this – partly as a result of the surgery (due to the crash nature I had an extra vertical incision made on my uterus to speed up the delivery, unbeknownst to me until a much later Birth Debrief, as it was invisible) – I have a great deal of scar tissue, and adhesions formed around the right side of my scar. This means I have long-term hip stiffness that needs ongoing attention through movement, massage and occasional physio/osteopathy. I could possibly have prevented it through massage.

Abdominal overhang

One of the potentially upsetting side-effects of your Caesarean birth will be that you have an overhang of your tummy above the scar site. How long this lasts is different for everyone. It's affected by your pre-baby muscle tone, the presence of adhesions, your postural habits, your pelvic organs 'shifting' within the pelvic cavity, the way your surgery was pinned. Too much activity or the wrong type of exercise too soon post Caesarean can also influence it happening. The only thing that will make a difference to this overhang is time, lots of patience, self-compassion and massage. It may never 'go back to normal', so an element of gentle acceptance is necessary.

Deep massage can help with your overhang by stimulating blood flow to the area and encouraging tone in the muscles. It also helps to break down abdominal tension that might be preventing your pelvic floor from functioning optimally. You might have numbness and lack of sensation around the scar site for quite a while. This can inhibit your abdominal and pelvic floor awareness. Massage also helps with this – anything that creates a mind–body connection will help to fire up pathways of sensation. I still have an overhang, and I continue to massage it every day, and I will do (whenever I remember) for as long as I'm living and moving.

Listen to your body. If you're still experiencing pain around your scar weeks and months after giving birth, go to your GP.

ABDOMINAL MASSAGE

Stage 1

We're trying to make the abdominal area as soft as butter, to enable your muscle awareness and engagement. This really influences your diaphragm and pelvic floor awareness and function.

- Lie on your back in Relaxation Position (*see* p. 56). Take your hands on to your tummy, or you can use a massage ball, such as a Yoga Tune Up ball, if you prefer. If you feel comfortable, begin to softly press all along the line of the linea alba, down the centre of your torso. Imagine you're *gently* kneading dough. Notice if there are any areas of tenderness or pain.

- Palpate around the ribs: take your fingertips around the bottom of the ribcage and trace the bottom of your ribs from your breastbone out and down. Focus gently on the area around the breastbone, which is one of the main areas where your diaphragm attaches.

- Breathe in and on the out-breath allow the tummy muscles to fully open and soften under your hands.

- Continue to palpate further down the tummy, around the ribcage, lower under the navel. Palpate the areas of tightness and tension.

- Just to the left of your navel, begin to knead a U shape, down below the navel – taking care towards your scar site – and then up to the right.

TIME'S A HEALER

Over time, your scar will stop being quite so red and angry, and will become more skin-coloured and may even fade away pretty much entirely. It all depends on your own birth story. For example, I have two Caesarean scars, in the same place. My firstborn's entrance into the world is characterised by a ragged and thick scar, which is dark in colour, uneven and slightly raised on one side. His was a panicked and rushed birth and the scar reflects this. My second is a gliding, tiny scar, which gleams its way in a perfect straight line through the ragged scar of my first. It's only just visible, more considered and calm than its predecessor – I had an elective Caesarean with my second. If that were my only scar, I might not even really see it any more.

HOW TO BOOST YOUR COLLAGEN LEVELS

Collagen is the main structural protein in connective tissue and as such is a very important element in postnatal recovery. It's worth noting that your collagen levels never rebuild to 100 per cent strength post abdominal surgery, so there will be some permanent marker of your experience in the healing power of your tissue, particularly if you have repeat surgery. Nevertheless, collagen strength can be optimised through your diet and hydration, so look to those pillars of self-care (rehydrate and refuel) in your recovery. This involves consuming lots of healing bone broth if you're not vegetarian, and generally optimising your protein intake for collagen rebuilding. Chicken soup really is profoundly healing. Other good sources are oily fish, cashew nuts, almonds, soy products and pulses.

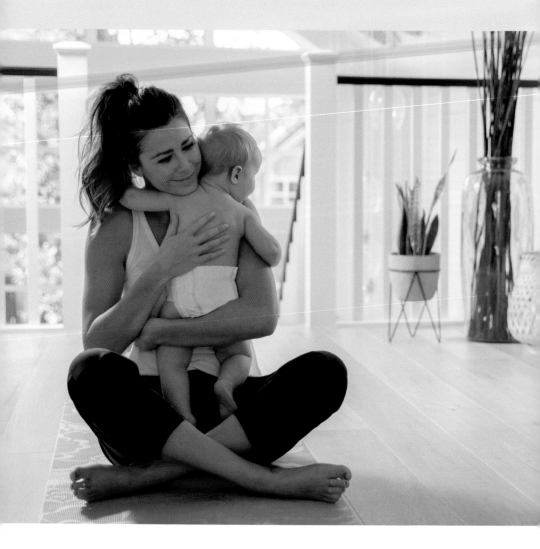

PELVIC TILTS PUSH WITH FEET
Stage 1

This exercise activates the core in a functional way, which aids load bearing – such as getting up from sitting and walking. It improves circulation and aids bowel function, which we can need a bit of help with post C-section. It can also take the focus away from an area that feels sore and vulnerable. We're used to Pelvic Tilts (*see* p. 57), but here using the feet as a driver creates a more functional stimulation for the pelvic floor and core muscles, and may change the way you experience the movement.

- Start in Relaxation Position (*see* p. 56).
- Breathe normally and slowly.
- Press the feet into the floor and allow the pelvis to tilt into the mat.

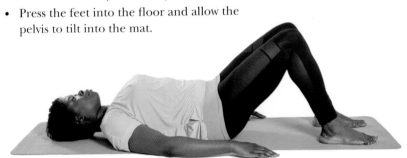

- Lengthen the torso to release the tailbone back down. Try to keep the buttocks soft and allow the heaviness of your pelvis to be unforced.

Myofascial lines

Caesarean birth has a profound impact on the 'Myofascial lines' of your body, as described by Thomas Myers in his wonderful book *Anatomy Trains* – that is, the connective tissue that carries interconnected movement messages around your body, from the soles of your feet to the crown of your head. Lines are severed, junctions are blocked, muscle awareness is diverted and disguised. Exactly like in a transport system, if there's a hold-up somewhere, a station is closed and a route is diverted, which will have a ripple effect somewhere else down the line and things won't run quite so smoothly for a bit – so it's to be expected that you may not feel 'the same' for a long time, maybe ever. But you can feel strong and energised again. You will strengthen your core.

SHOULDER DROPS, FLY BREATHS
Stage 1

We need to release tension around the neck and shoulder area, and this is a great way to do it. It's also good for establishing correct postural habits and shoulder alignment for when you're carrying your baby.

- Lie in Relaxation Position (*see* p. 56). Lengthen your arms up towards the ceiling, shoulder-width apart, palms facing each other.

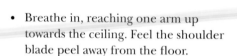

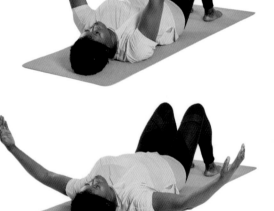

- Breathe in, reaching one arm up towards the ceiling. Feel the shoulder blade peel away from the floor.

- Breathe out and soften the arm down, allowing the shoulder joint to release fully down on to the floor.

- Repeat up to 10 times on each arm.

- Breathe in to open your arms out to the sides. Imagine your ribcage opening wide, too.

- Breathe out as you close them towards each other, softening the ribs into your torso.

- Repeat 5–10 times.

Watchpoints

Sighing the breath out ('haaaaaa') lets you find a 'ragdoll' feeling around the shoulder.

Try to keep the head, pelvis and spine still.

WINDMILL ARMS

Stage 1

This tones your arms, offering a wonderful release across the chest and shoulders. It's also great for clearing your mind, as you have to focus on coordination.

Stage 2

Optional equipment: hand weights up to 1.5kg (3lb)

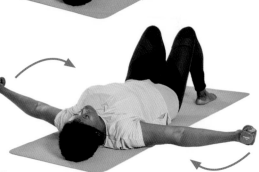

- Align yourself in Relaxation Position (*see* p. 56) (optional: holding a weight in each hand). Lengthen both arms above you, shoulder-width apart, palms facing forwards.
- Breathe in and lengthen through the spine.

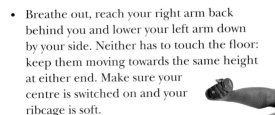

- Breathe out, reach your right arm back behind you and lower your left arm down by your side. Neither has to touch the floor: keep them moving towards the same height at either end. Make sure your centre is switched on and your ribcage is soft.

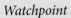

- Breathe in and circle your arms outstretched along the floor to bring the arms to opposite ends of the body.

- Return both arms to the start position. Maintain a heavy ribcage.
- Breathe out and reverse the direction.
- Repeat up to 5 times in each direction.

> *Watchpoint*
> Your neck should be relaxed, with a space between the shoulders and your ears.

RIBCAGE CLOSURE WITH LEG EXTENSION
Stage 1

This exercise challenges your coordination and your pelvic and spinal stability. It's a great one for balancing the mind by focusing on the timing of the movement, being able to control the flowing movement of your arms and legs at the same pace. We need to keep the torso heavy and stable, while the limbs move freely and without tension.

- Align yourself in Relaxation Position (*see* p. 56) holding a band shoulder width between your hands.

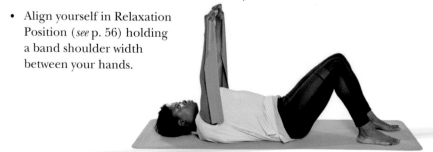

- Breathe in to lengthen and prepare for movement.
- Breathe out and release your arms back behind you towards the floor – they may remain level with your ears. Simultaneously, slide the right leg away along the floor, in line with your hip. Check that your torso is stable and the ribcage remains soft.

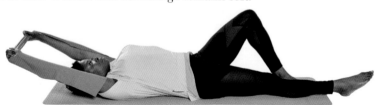

- Breathe in, lengthen the limbs away from your centre, without allowing the back to arch and the ribcage to 'pop' to the ceiling.
- Breathe out to return to the start position.
- Repeat up to 10 times, alternating legs.

Watchpoints

Imagine your torso as a rectangle from shoulder to hips and try to maintain that stable shape throughout the movement; keep the shoulders open and relaxed and the pelvis still.

Keep the lower ribs softened, as though tucked into your trousers.

Make sure your leg slides directly in line with your hip, not out to the side or in towards the other leg.

TWISTING SPINE CURL
Stage 2

This is a variation on the Spine Curl (*see* p. 82), working into a full circumduction (all movements) of the spine, which feels like a great massage and unknots some tension in your spine. It can be a great way of discovering imbalances you didn't realise you had. (Easy to do even with a baby draped across you, I promise.)

- Start as for Spine Curls (*see* p. 82).
- Breathe out and roll your weight on to your left hip.

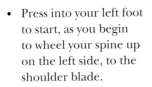

- Press into your left foot to start, as you begin to wheel your spine up on the left side, to the shoulder blade.

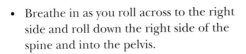

- Breathe in as you roll across to the right side and roll down the right side of the spine and into the pelvis.

- Continue to roll in this direction 4 times, then reverse the direction.

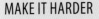

MAKE IT HARDER
Add a little more challenge by raising the arms up towards the ceiling as you roll through the spine. Keep your ribcage soft and an appropriate connection to your centre.

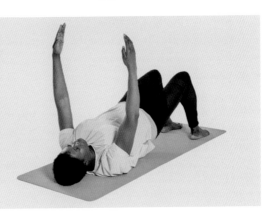

BAND RAISE
Stage 2

This exercise releases tightness around your pectorals (chest muscles) and corrects your posture. It's also great for making you aware of your rib–hip placement, which is so important for waking up your core muscles between your ribcage and pelvis.

• Align yourself in High Kneeling – on your knees, lifting your spine upright – on your mat, or standing. Hold the ends of a stretchy band, or a scarf, in each hand.

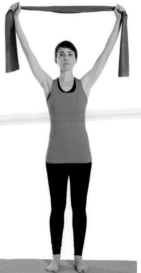

• Breathe in. Connect to your centre and float your arms forwards and up, reaching the band above your head.

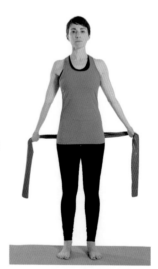

• Breathe in and reach the arms back behind you, without bending the arms. If this is too challenging and you can't do it without moving your head, adjust the position of your hands to hold the band slightly wider.

• Breathe out, lengthen the right arm back over the head, in front to shoulder height.
  Breathing normally, lengthen the left arm over.

• Release the arms back down.

• Repeat up to 6 times.

Watchpoints

Do this in front of a mirror so you can be sure of your technique.

Keep your head upright: avoid popping your head forwards like a pigeon when your band comes above your head.

Soften your shoulders and try not to allow them to hunch up to your ears.

Make sure that your back isn't arching as you raise the arms.

SITTING CROSS-LEGGED ROLL FORWARD
Stage 1

This explores the idea of forward flexion, stretching into the back of your body and gently waking up your abdominal muscles without load. You can use a small Pilates ball, or a foam roller (or even a child's football!).

- Sit cross-legged, tall on your sit bones. Place a small ball on the floor in front of your shins: it's good if it's slightly deflated so that you can soften your palms evenly into the ball. Breathe in and lengthen up, relaxing the arms.

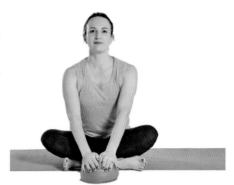

- Breathe out and roll the ball forwards, keeping your arms and upper body lengthening and reaching away with positive energy as far as you comfortably can, lifting gently into your centre.

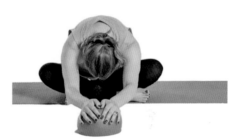

- Breathe in and feel the back of the body stretching. Then roll yourself back, with control.
- Repeat 3 times, then cross the legs the other way (other leg in front) and repeat 3 more times.
- As a variation, you can then roll the ball on a diagonal to each side, making sure you also change the cross of your legs evenly. Keep the torso stable and your sit bones heavy into the mat.

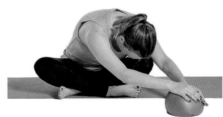

TYPEWRITER RIBS EXTENDED ARMS
Stage 1

This is a wonderful way of encouraging *awareness* of the alignment of your ribs and hips. It's also great for stimulating healing for diastasis recti and of creating awareness of the oblique muscles of the waist – perfect for counterbalancing the mum hunch. It is so called because the ribcage slides in the horizontal like a typewriter, rather than tipping like a teapot. (You do remember typewriters, right…?)

- Stand against a wall. Place your hands on the sides of your ribcage. Feel the shoulder blades softly open against the wall. The spine is in neutral with the natural curves lengthened. Knees softly bent.

- On an out-breath, lengthen your torso to the left, leading with the left fingertips. Lean directly to the left as if your ribcage is a typewriter sliding above your pelvis. This isn't a Side Reach (*see* p. 64) to the diagonal tipping like a teapot, but instead moving the ribcage in parallel with the pelvis below it, like a vintage typewriter sliding above the keyboard, keeping the pelvis stable.

- Breathe in to return, then breathe out and reach to the right.
- Keep your shoulder blades wide, and shoulders level.

VARIATION

For more massage into the shoulder joints, take your standing position away from the wall (you could also do this sitting down), and add a twist into the shoulder joints: as you reach to the right, rotate both arms from the shoulder through to the wrist/fingertips, as if spiralling from your wrist out to the opposite arm, like wringing a cloth.

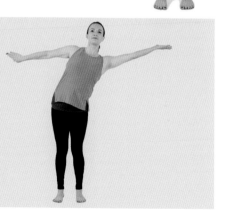

STANDING WALL PUSH-UP
Stage 2

The wall is a brilliant resource for our recovery – there's always one around, and you can use it in those moments at home while you're making a cup of tea, etc.

This exercise encourages your abdominal strength without the load of a horizontal push-up. You could also do it against the counter top in the kitchen. To increase the challenge, step further away from the wall. To make it easier, come closer.

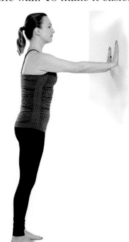

- Stand tall, arm's length away from the wall, with your palms released wide into the wall. Adjust your foot position to make sure you are comfortable.
- Breathe in to lengthen into the spine.

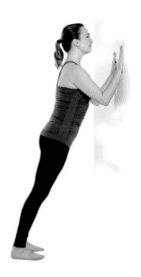

- Breathe out and push forwards into the wall, bending your elbows in towards your waist rather than out to the side. Your body should move as one connected unit, spine and hips. You may feel a nice stretch in the calf muscles.
- Breathe in and lengthen away. Repeat up to 10 times.

VARIATION

This is a great stretch for any mothering day, to stretch the upper back and open the shoulders – you can even do this using your buggy as a support.

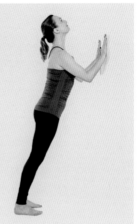

- To make it more challenging: as you push forwards, nod your nose up, to open the chest into a wall Cobra. The extension should be from your breastbone, felt in your mid-spine around the bra-strap area, and not into the lower spine. Keep your abdominals lifted.
- To finish, stick your bottom out and reach your arms forwards into the wall, to come into a standing Downward Dog.

MODIFIED PUSH-UP
Stage 2

A more challenging exercise – only attempt it once you feel comfortable in your abdominal connection. This strengthens your chest and shoulders, adds more challenge for your core control. Great for doing while you're playing on the floor with baby.
Push up to a kiss!

- Start in Four-point Kneeling (*see* p. 77). Lengthen into your neutral spine.
- Take a few moments to breathe abdominally, softening your belly on the in-breath and lifting your abdominals on the out-breath, to connect to your centre.

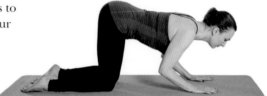

- On an in-breath, bend your elbows to lower your chest down between your hands. Keep the spine neutral.

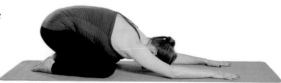

- As you breathe out, press back up to Four-point Kneeling.
- Repeat up to 10 times, then release back into Rest Position (*see* p. 81).

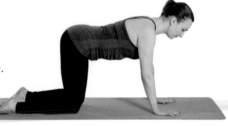

VARIATION
Stage 3

This is a much more challenging version. When you feel like you want to judge your stability and strength, add a lift of the leg, taking care not to arch your back. If this is too much, come back to **Stage 2** and try again when you've focused on deeper awareness and connection. The great thing about this exercise is that it challenges you in a slightly unbalanced position – in motherhood, we are rarely evenly loaded in our day-to-day lives: often carrying scooters, car seats and babies on one side rather than the other. We need to train our body in a way that mirrors our daily function – which will highlight where you might have weakness and imbalances that need to be addressed.

- In Four-point Kneeling (*see* p. 77) lengthen one leg away from you, as for Table Top Leg Extend (*see* p. 103).
- On an out-breath, reach your leg to hip height.

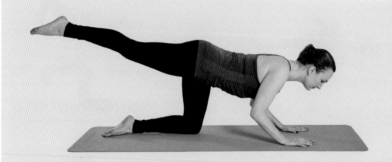

- As you breathe in, lower into a push-up, as you reach the leg in line with the spine.
- Lower the leg, but keep it extended. Repeat with the same leg 5 times, then release back into Rest Position (*see* p. 81) before repeating on the other side.

CAESAREAN RECOVERY WORKOUTS

5-minute workout	
Relaxation: Pelvic Floor: Pubic Bone Breathing 102	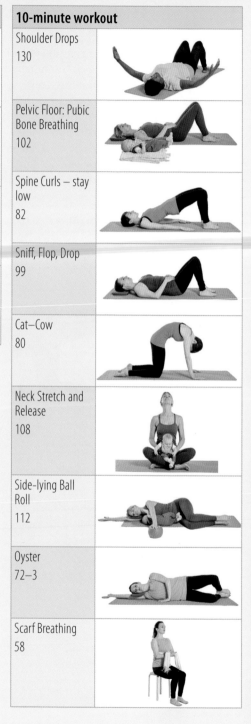
Pelvic Tilts Push with Feet 129	
Windmill Arms 131	
Hip Flexor Stretch 109	

10-minute workout	
Shoulder Drops 130	
Pelvic Floor: Pubic Bone Breathing 102	
Spine Curls – stay low 82	
Sniff, Flop, Drop 99	
Cat–Cow 80	
Neck Stretch and Release 108	
Side-lying Ball Roll 112	
Oyster 72–3	
Scarf Breathing 58	

CAESAREAN RECOVERY WORKOUTS

20-minute workout		20-minute workout cont.	
Relaxation: Pelvic Floor: Pubic Bone Breathing 102		Typewriter Ribs 136	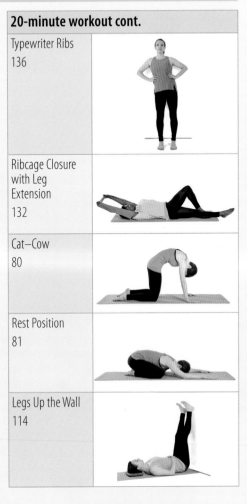
Pelvic floor awareness exercises 99		Ribcage Closure with Leg Extension 132	
Knee Drops 69		Cat–Cow 80	
Compass 75–6		Rest Position 81	
Band Raise 134		Legs Up the Wall 114	
Sitting Cross-legged Roll 135			
Twisting Spine Curl 133			

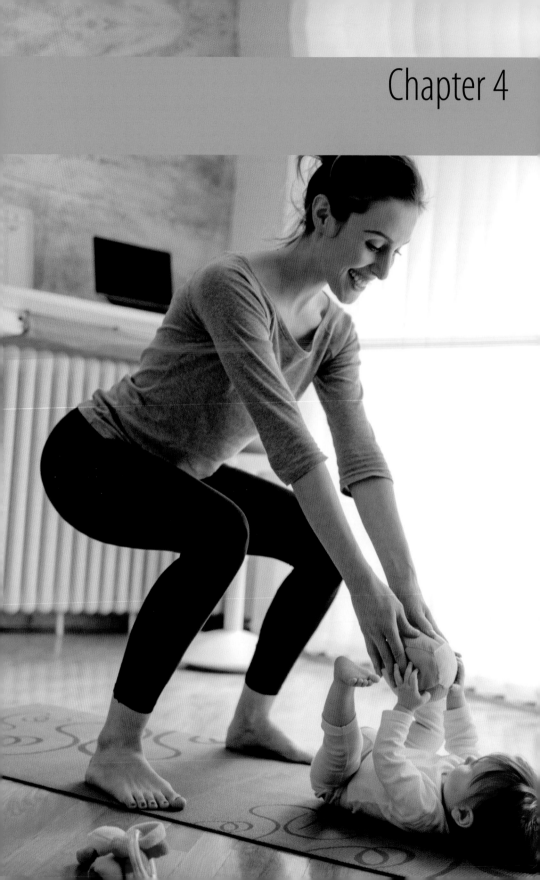

Chapter 4

Building up your strength: 'nine months in, nine months out'

The six months beyond the fourth trimester brings huge changes for your baby: the transition from relatively passive, sleepy* and portable newborn to a fully fledged, moving, communicating, rapidly unfolding and demanding personality. The phrase 'nine months in, nine months out' is used as an encouraging way of saying that you built your baby for nine months, so you should look to that full period after your baby has left the premises to gradually 'get back to the way you were': whether that's 'shedding baby weight' or feeling fitter and stronger, 'your old self'. * *(NB no eye rolls if that wasn't your experience, it wasn't mine either first time round – he was very cranky, neither passive nor sleepy...)*

I definitely prefer this angle to the idea that you should be back in your 'pre-pregnancy jeans' (or modelling on the catwalk, thanks Heidi Klum) two weeks after birth, but I still feel that nine months is the blink of an eye postnatally for some of us and we should always look at ourselves as new, today, rather than trying to 'get back' to what we may have been before. In this six months after your fourth trimester, you are hopefully feeling 'more normal' and slightly more used to catering to the daily (and nightly) demands of a small person, and your energy levels may be beginning to rise. Any pelvic floor and diastasis recti issues may be feeling stronger and perhaps 'fixed'. But equally ... you may be wandering around in a zombie state, sighing about how tired you are, wishing your baby would sleep more ... while simultaneously wondering where on earth the time has gone and deeply feeling you want to press pause and keep them from growing so fast. If you have a particularly sleepless baby/babies and/or have had no time to devote to mothering yourself, you might be feeling heavy and exhausted. Remember, lack of sleep/rest inhibits the healing process, so an element of depletion, fatigue and weakness is to be expected if you're not getting any real rest.

Intense fatigue a few months in may be purely due to your beautiful little sleep vampire, or it could be related to something else – it's worth investigating thyroid issues or iron deficiency (anaemia) for example at this stage to rule that out, if it's a full-body type of fatigue that you've never experienced before. And, mental health flags – fatigue and depletion can have an impact on your emotional resilience, so be aware of your inner landscape. You may well have lost loads of weight and be in your pre-pregnancy jeans but still suffering from incontinence, which shows that although you've 'bounced back', your insides are still not fully healed. You may have ongoing weakness in your core, or pelvic organ prolapse, which means your rehab journey is looking like an extended one – it truly depends on *you* and your own personal postnatal experience. There is no 'you should be feeling ... at this stage' to judge yourself against. Meet yourself where you are now.

In this six-month period the pressure to be 'feeling fine' is strong. Take it at *your* pace and don't compare yourself to other mums – particularly not on social media. Physiologically, your systems will most likely have settled down by now and the hormonal fluctuation is minimal once your periods have returned. But there is *always* flux in our female cycles so it's worth noticing when your cycle settles down to be even or regular once it has returned. And if it doesn't, investigate with your GP why this might be. If you're still breastfeeding, the scientific jury is out as to whether this impacts on your ligament strength beyond the first couple of months. I prefer to err on the side of caution to say that it possibly does, and that it's a good idea to look after yourself with that in mind: try to take it easy with the HIIT and dynamic yoga if you're breastfeeding. Even if you're not, your menstrual cycle has an effect on your propensity to injury. Hormones may have an impact on prolapse symptoms, for example oestrogen dip may increase severity so just before your period you may find that symptoms are more apparent. It's key not to see your recovery as linear: some weeks you may feel weaker than others. There will be times when you need to preserve energy, and others when you feel you're raring to go. Try not to get frustrated, but instead piece it together by tracking how *you* feel on *your* cycle, and plan accordingly.

If you're still breastfeeding (undoubtedly a wonderful thing beyond the first six months but, obviously, no judgement if you're not and never did), it physically continues to deplete your energies so keep track of your water intake and optimise your diet in just the same way as you hopefully could in the fourth trimester.

Babies only get heavier, so at this stage you're placing increasing, more repetitive pressure on your pelvic floor, abdominals, neck, shoulders and knees constantly lifting, carrying, and getting up and down from the floor as you play with your ever-more mobile and 'into everything' baby. You might be returning to work and into that adult world of desks and juggling stress. Your core needs to be strong to make sure you don't succumb to aches and pains (it's in this period and the early toddler time with both my children that I injured my knee and shoulder – both due to lack of deep core strength and sleep, and the general pack horse demands of small babies, so it's a real hotspot in the postnatal healing process). You

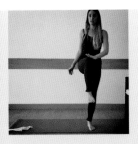

EXPERT ADVICE

Jo Diplock, PT and Pilates teacher specialising in Motherhood Core Restore, and mum of two

The biggest thing to remember is that your body has undergone a massive journey and change. Your organs will spend the nine months after birth reshuffling themselves back into their original positions. It's never been a more important time to be kind to yourself and not succumb to pressures of an exercise workload that's too progressive for the level your body is at.

Meet your body where it is now, and using Pilates and breath work you'll be able to lay solid foundations for getting back into full fitness and strength. House foundations are made from concrete, which needs time to set and can never be rushed – that's exactly the approach you need to take. Reconnecting, re-educating in a lot of parts and rehabbing your body one step at a time.

Symptoms of weakness – achy back, knees or leaking pelvic floor – are your body's way of telling you it's not strong enough for the level you are living life or training at. Never ignore those symptoms. The joy of Pilates and breath connection work is that you'll heal all the deep core muscles and maybe even come back stronger than you were before.

www.themotherhoodmovement.com
Instagram @the_motherhood_movement
Facebook https://www.facebook.com/themotherhoodmovementofficial/

need to release the tension of all the additional weightlifting you're doing day to day.

In this six-month period we'll venture more into **Stage 3** territory. But we'll continue to revisit **Stages 1** and **2**. Be *curious* about your strength and how your body–mind is coping with motherhood. Postnatal recovery isn't linear and you might find that in the six months after your baby emerges beyond 'newborn' you feel totally amazing and 'back to normal', full of energy and feeling great … but also you could feel even weaker than during the initial postnatal period, which can make you feel frustrated, depleted and low. This is to be expected with the cumulative depletion of sleep, of breastfeeding, and responding to your baby's ever-changing needs and demands.

Check in with the four pillars: *Rest, Rehydrate, Refuel, Revitalise.* Look at where you are within your own personal progress framework: **Stage 1, 2** … now ready for **3**?

Posture tips for your changing shape

Revisit the posture tips on p. 52–4 regularly to notice your patterns of movement and your lifting technique. It's these, rather than any 'exercise' that you might be doing, that put the most pressure on your pelvic floor and core muscles every day. Notice whether you're beginning to carry your baby on the same side whenever you pick her up. Notice whether you have any *awareness* of engaging strength in your centre when you are putting him in the car seat, or lifting her out of the bath. If not, commit to checking in with that more regularly.

The buggy is a good trigger for reminding you to do so. Use the buggy handles: place your hands on the handle/s and exert a bit of pressure down into your hands while standing strong into your feet, to encourage you to soften your shoulders and stand tall. Do the Back Stretch Against the Buggy/Wall (*see* p. 65), some Pliés (*see* p. 88) or Squats (*see* p. 154–6) and a calf stretch whenever you find yourself standing still. Feel your shoulders soften into your back and your heart centre lift. Grow tall like a sunflower. Often, we'll push the buggy with one hand and scroll on our phones with the other. This multitasking is doing our bodies (and spirit) no favours.

The Mummy MOT

Now is a great time to have a check-up with a women's health physio if you haven't already. Your initial stage of automatic healing has completed and now it's up to you to take more responsibility for things going the way you want them to in terms of your strength and resilience. Remember, postnatal issues don't just disappear if ignored. A client recently contacted me to begin postnatal core restore classes. Her 'baby' is now three and she was 'hoping her diastasis recti would have gone away by now' – healing doesn't work that way sadly: not when you're lifting ever-increasing weights every day but not adapting your posture or deep strength.

Maybe the newborn fog has lifted and you're keen to pay more attention to your pelvic floor and core. Go to your GP as a first port of call to ask to be referred to a physio. If you can, invest privately in an assessment.

I've included details in the Resources for places to go for further information about women's health physiotherapy and how to find a practitioner near you.

BUILDING UP YOUR STRENGTH

Your baby is getting bigger and more mobile. So, let's get strengthening.

CURL-UPS
Stage 3

If you're getting yourself out of bed every day, picking up your baby, lifting the car seat, pushing your buggy, *you're using your abdominals*. A gentle Curl-up, performed with care and conscious breathing, creates less intra-abdominal pressure (load on your pelvic floor/pull on your diastasis recti) than getting up from the floor or lifting a heavyweight toddler. So, although we need to proceed with caution, it's an important part of your healing toolkit. Wait for 12 weeks post Caesarean before making this a regular part of your workouts, or at least until you have no tenderness in the scar area and you feel you can recruit your pelvic floor (or have been checked by a physio).

Curl-ups ask you to find your X Factor – Body Control Pilates® describes the X factor as your rib-to-opposite-hip connection, an imaginary X across your body connecting your muscle energy together.

- Lie in Relaxation Position (*see* p. 56). Place your hands behind your head.

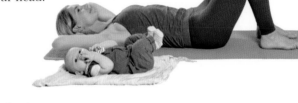

- Breathe in and lengthen the back of the neck. Keep your head on the floor but tuck your chin to your chest.
- Breathe out and draw in and up into your pelvic floor and lower abdominals. Begin to lift your head and the upper back off the mat.

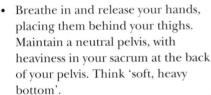

- Breathe in and release your hands, placing them behind your thighs. Maintain a neutral pelvis, with heaviness in your sacrum at the back of your pelvis. Think 'soft, heavy bottom'.

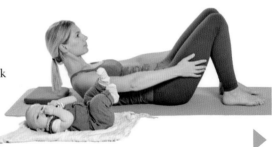

- Breathe out and gently hold on behind the thighs to support you lifting a few more segments off the mat.

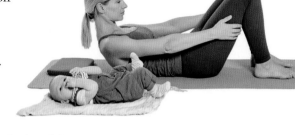

- Breathe in to release the hands back behind the head.
- Breathe out to lower back down with control.
- Repeat 5 times.

*If you see any doming in your abdominals or feel pressure in the pelvic floor – come back to try this later after you've continued with your **Stage 2** deep core work.*

CURL-UPS WITH LEG SLIDE

Stage 3

This is a great way of really finding the deep core connection and awareness of your pelvic stability.

- Start in Curl-ups position (*see* p. 147).
- Breathe in to prepare. On an out-breath, curl up with control. Simultaneously, slide your leg away, as for Leg Slides (p. 68).

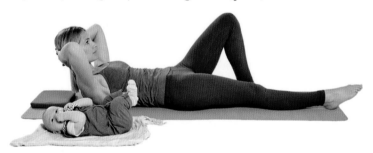

- Breathe in and lower back down, as you glide the leg back in. Repeat up to 5 times on each leg.

Watchpoint

Control any movement of the pelvis with your deep core engagement.

DOUBLE KNEE FOLDS
Stage 3

This requires core control and abdominal strength. We need to deeply recruit pelvic floor and abdominals properly to control the movement and ensure that there is *no doming*. If there is doming, or you can't prevent your pelvis from tilting/your back from arching, this exercise is too much for you *right now* so you need to bring it back to **Stage 1 Awareness**. Practise Single Knee Folds (*see* p. 71) until you have the required deep strength.

- Breathe in to prepare.
- Breathe out, float one knee in as for Single Knee Folds (*see* p. 71). Try to maintain neutral spine and pelvis.

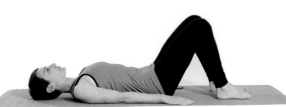

- On the same breath, deepen your connection to your centre, float the second leg in. If you need to, consciously tuck the pelvis and imprint your lower spine for support.

  Make it a conscious movement rather than a result of the weight of the legs tipping your pelvis.

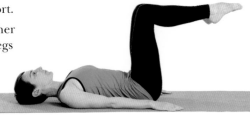

- Breathe in, soften the shoulders and relax your torso.

- Breathe out, stay connected to your centre as you float the first foot back down, followed by the second.
- Repeat up to 5 times.

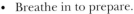

Watchpoint
Try not to *brace* the body: there should be ease of movement.

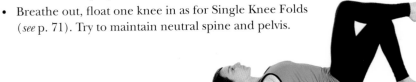

BACK RELEASE OVER ROLLER
Stage 2

The foam roller is such a fabulous piece of kit for mums. This exercise really gets into those upper-back tense knots that babies and children create, plus it requires balance and control so we're gently working our deep core muscles, too. If you don't have a foam roller, I'd advise getting hold of one as even just lying your spine along the roller counteracts the mum hunch and stimulates core engagement. If not, you can simulate this by placing a small ball in between your shoulder blades, or even placing two tennis balls underneath your shoulder blade area.

- Place the roller on your mat. Sit down in front of it and then with control release yourself back so that your shoulder blades are balanced on the roller. Take your hands behind your head and release your bum down into the mat, knees bent. Breathe in to lengthen the spine and soften your ribcage into your torso.

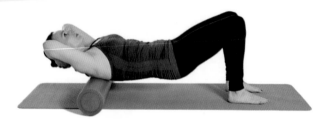

- Breathe out and lift your bum in line with your ribs. Breathing normally, roll your upper body slowly, forwards and back. Massage into the upper spine – maintaining neutral rather than doing any arching and tucking.

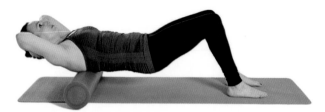

- Gently release your bottom back to the floor and roll yourself off the roller.

HIP FLEXOR BOW AND ARROW
Stage 3

This exercise challenges your balance and stretches the hip and shoulder area. Quite a lot of core work is required to keep you stable, but it's low impact. If it's too much, you can do exactly the same movement from High Kneeling.

- Come into a high Lunge as for upright Hip Flexor Stretch (*see* p. 109), then bring your right knee forwards. Release your weight with control forwards over your front knee, to open into the left hip. Lengthen both arms out in front of you at shoulder height. Relax the shoulders, your palms facing each other.

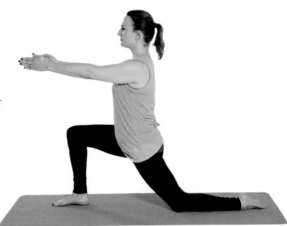

- Bend your elbow and draw back the left arm, twisting your spine to follow the movement. Straighten the arm and reach it back behind you, looking back. Open into your left hip as you stretch the chest.

- Float the arm back to centre. Repeat 5 times on this side, then swap to the other side.

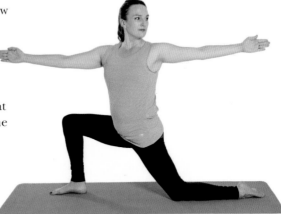

> *Watchpoint*
> Make sure you aren't arching your back. Maintain a strong centre all the time.

SIDE-LYING ELBOW TO KNEE
Stages 2–3

This exercise is brilliant for strengthening the oblique muscles and honing your coordination, working on the strength of your hips and bum. The aim is to keep your torso and spine long and stable while the limbs move. It's slightly more dynamic and fast paced than some of the other exercises, so will get your blood flowing a bit more.

- Begin lying on your side, with your arm outstretched and a pillow in between your head and your arm. Bend your legs in to 90 degrees, your spine long and in neutral.

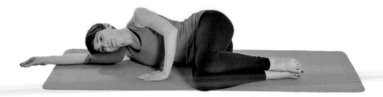

Breathe in to lengthen and prepare for movement, then breathe out to release your top arm up and over your head, and your top leg out in line with your hip.

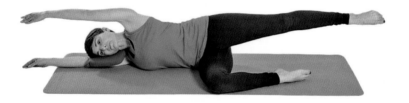

- On an out-breath, bend your top arm and knee in towards each other, then breathe in to release them away with control.

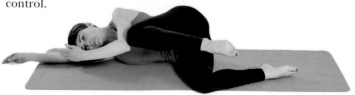

- Repeat 10 times.
- Finish by stretching the top arm and the top leg away, relaxing them on to the floor and breathe into the length of the top side of the waist. Then either move to another side-lying exercise, or move on to the other side.

MAKE IT HARDER

This is a much more challenging version that needs more core strength, balance and control.

Stage 3

- Come into a supported Side Plank position: from High Kneeling, reach your right arm down to the floor. Then reach your left arm up above your head in a diagonal and the left leg away from the body in the same diagonal. Breathe in to lengthen.

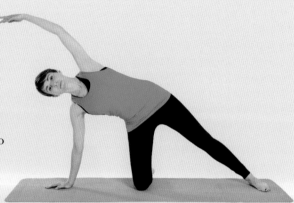

- On an out-breath, bend the top arm and leg in towards each other, above your waist. Stay lifted and strong in your centre. Reach them away to the start position as you breathe in.

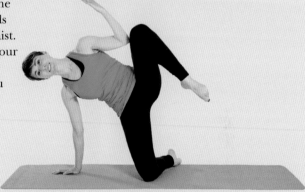

- Repeat 10 times. Finish by releasing into Rest Position (*see* p. 81), before changing sides.

SQUAT WITH ARM CIRCLE
Stage 3

Squats are a brilliantly functional Pilates exercise. You're squatting 1700 times a day with small babies and children anyway, so let's make it count. Take care if you are still suffering from pelvic floor dysfunction or pelvic organ prolapse. Deep squats place quite a load into your pelvic floor so you must take care to hinge properly into your hip joints, rather than tucking the pelvis underneath you as you bend. *If you feel any sensation of bearing down in your vagina, avoid this exercise and seek advice from your physio.*

This version of the Squat helps you to learn to stabilise your pelvis, challenges your balance, opens your shoulders and strengthens your thighs, hips, knees and ankles.

- Stand, arms relaxed by your sides, palms facing in towards your thighs.

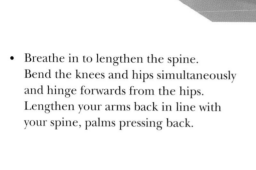

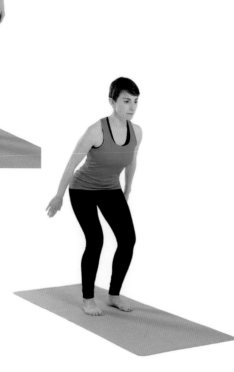

- Breathe in to lengthen the spine. Bend the knees and hips simultaneously and hinge forwards from the hips. Lengthen your arms back in line with your spine, palms pressing back.

- Breathe out and straighten through the backs of the legs to stand upright once more, simultaneously floating the arms forwards and up above the head.

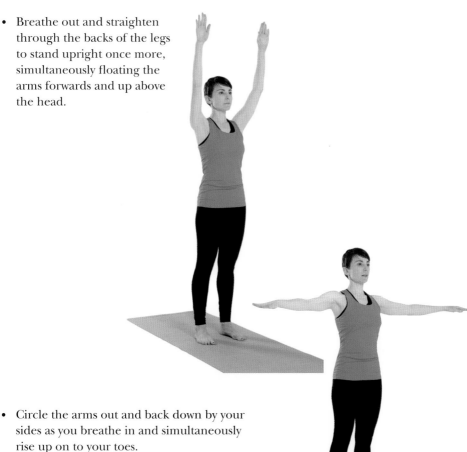

- Circle the arms out and back down by your sides as you breathe in and simultaneously rise up on to your toes.

- Lower your heels with control, back to the start position.

- Repeat up to 10 times.

Watchpoints

Imagine a pole resting down the back of your body as you squat: head, shoulders, lower back. Make sure you are sticking your bottom directly behind you, rather than tucking your pelvis under. Think long tail.

Only lower as far as you can comfortably lift yourself back up again.

Keep the hips, knees and ankles parallel.

Imagine the crown of the head and the tailbone lengthening away from each other.

STANDING CAT WITH WINDMILL ARMS
Stages 2–3

This exercise gives you a great feedback for where your spine and
pelvis are in space, which will help you gauge your posture day to
day. It works your core strongly but in a supported position, and
encourages flexible shoulders. You can also do this without
the arm movement, resting the hands on your thighs.

- Standing tall, hinge forwards into a Squat.
- Take one hand on to your pelvis, palm facing out, the
  other palm behind your head. Lengthen your spine
  into neutral and actively connect the back of the head
  into the hand.

- Breathe in to lengthen, as you
  breathe out, tuck your tailbone
  underneath you and roll your
  spine into a standing Cat
  (*see* p. 80).

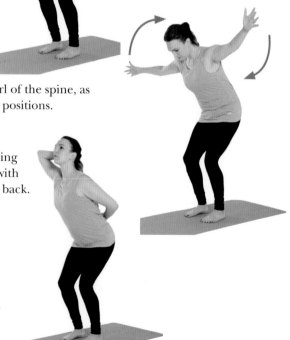

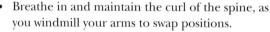

- Breathe in and maintain the curl of the spine, as
  you windmill your arms to swap positions.

- Breathe out and uncurl, extending
  into a standing Cow (*see* p. 80) with
  a gentle extension of the upper back.
  Windmill your arms back.

- Breathe in to return to neutral.
- Repeat 6–10 times.

ROLL-BACKS WITH BAND
Stages 2–3

This exercise is perfect for strengthening the deep abdominals without too much load, so it's suitable for any diastasis recti. If you see any doming at all, remain at a lengthened active C-curve (**Stage 2**) rather than rolling back, until you can control the load and your deep supporting muscles can support you enough. You can do this without a band, either resting your hands lightly behind your thighs, or lengthen them out in front of you in line with your shoulders (which is harder).

- Sitting tall in your sit bones, lengthen the legs out in front of you and loop a band around your feet, taking one end in each hand. Soften the knees, heels down into the floor, toes up.

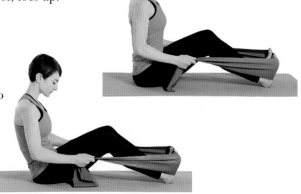

- Breathe in to lengthen tall. As you breathe out, connect to your centre and tuck your tailbone underneath you, lengthening into a C-curve.

- Either stay here, or, release your C-curve back, holding softly on to the band, elbows bent.

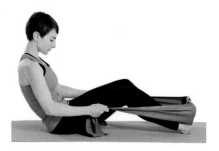

- Breathe in to lengthen and stay engaged into your centre as you maintain the position.
- Breathe out to roll your C-curve forwards, then roll up on to your sit bones, back into neutral.

Watchpoints

Keep the shoulders relaxed, try not to let them creep up to your ears.

Avoid slumping back – this is an active lifting curve, so maintain a strong centre, feeling opposing length between the crown of the head and tailbone.

Try to avoid 'gripping' with the hip flexors – your strength comes from deep within your pelvic floor and lower abdominals.

▶

MAKE IT HARDER

Stage 3

When you can definitely manage your abdominal strength with no doming, you can add more challenge with a rotation.

- When you are curled back, stay curled and bend your elbow to open your band out to one side, turning your torso to that side. Feel your waist muscles working to support your torso.

- Return to centre, then bring your C-curve forwards and release back to neutral.

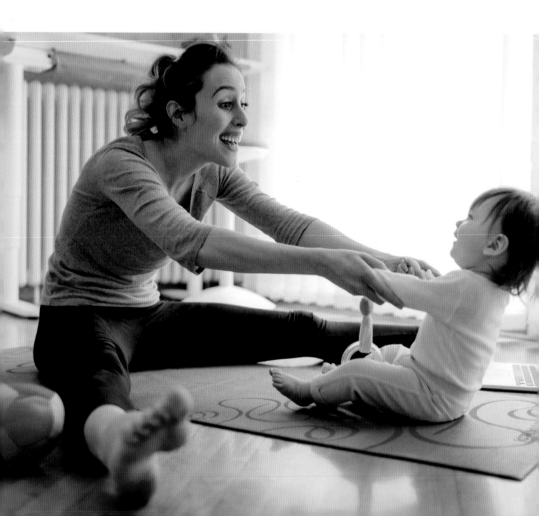

TABLE TOP LIFT AND LOWER
Stage 3

This exercise challenges the stability of your spine and shoulders, moving your limbs, developing your proprioception (sense of body placement and movement) and balance.

- Start in Four-point Kneeling (*see* p. 77). Imagine you have a tray of champagne balanced on your bottom.
- Breathe in, lengthen the spine.

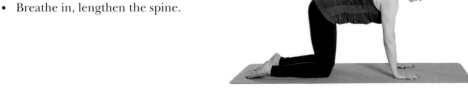

- Breathe out. Keeping your tray of champagne balanced, slide one leg out behind you, in line with your hip. Keep the foot in contact with the mat. At the same time, release the opposite arm away along the floor in front of you, in line with your shoulder, keeping the fingers in contact with the mat.

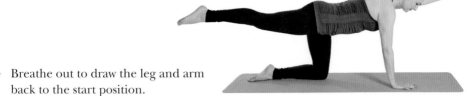

- Breathe in and maintain this lengthened position. Try not to allow your spine to waver and dip on one side – you'll spill your tray!
- Breathe out and lift the arm and leg to hip height. Then lower. Repeat 5 times on the same leg.

- Breathe out to draw the leg and arm back to the start position.
- Repeat up to 5 times on each side.

Watchpoint

Ensure you're not hip dipping – as you draw the leg back in it should slide back without you having to adjust the height of your pelvis.

MERMAID WITH TWIST
Stage 3

This is a more challenging one for your core. It's also a lovely hip opener and a stretch into the waist and upper back.

- Unusually for Pilates, this exercise begins in an asymmetrical position. Sitting tall with crossed legs, bring your right leg back behind you so your legs create a 'fan' shape. Try to ensure that you can sit evenly on your sit bones rather than slumping to one side – maybe take a pillow or a small ball underneath one sit bone if it's raised. You want to be able to lift evenly out of the hips, so that your shoulders are even, not tilted.

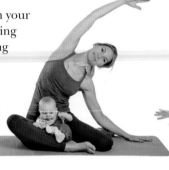

- Breathe in to reach your right arm up, keeping your left arm resting on your left shin. Breathing out, lift up and out of your waist to reach your right arm over in a diagonal.

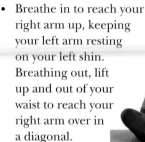
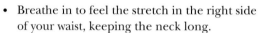

- Breathe in to feel the stretch in the right side of your waist, keeping the neck long.
- Breathe out as you lengthen back to centre and reach the left arm up and over to the left, reaching your right arm on to the floor. Take a breath in here.

- Then, as you breathe out, lower the left arm along the floor and twist your upper body to face the mat, bringing both arms out towards the mat. Breathe in here.

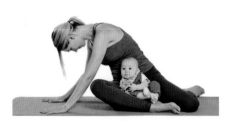

- Breathe out, strongly connecting to your core as you rise back to centre. Repeat 3 more times either side.
- Repeat, with the legs in a different cross.

Watchpoint

When you're reaching across, keep the underside of your waist active and lifted.

BABY COBRA WITH NECK ROLL AND TWIST
Stage 2

Your baby will have done exactly this extension when you first introduced him to tummy time, learning to lift the weight of his head away from the floor. You're both working the same deep stabilising postural muscles. This also gives you a great massage for your hips and lower spine. You can do just the upper body movement, without taking the rotation into the legs, if it is too challenging.

- Begin on your front, your forehead released on to a small pillow. Bend your elbows and open your arms out by your sides, with your hands in line with your forehead, palms facing down. Make sure there's a comfortable space between your elbows and your waist. Your wrists are in line with your elbows, not pressing in towards your shoulders. Ensure your collarbones feel open and wide. Your legs are slightly wider than hip width and turned out.

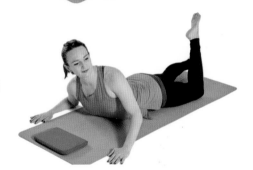

- Breathe in to prepare.
- Breathe out, look towards your left shoulder, and begin to peel your chest off the mat, straightening the left arm. Open the throat without overextending your neck. The bottom of your ribcage stays connected to the mat, right arm softly pressing into the floor.

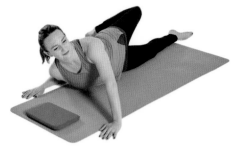

- As you open the spine and straighten the left arm, bend the left knee and begin to lift the leg off the mat. Twist the hips to dip the right toe across the right side.

- Breathe out and release your leg and hips back to centre and lower your chest back down, rolling the upper spine sequentially, as you did for a Spine Curl (*see* p. 82).
- Repeat up to 5 times on each side, then release back into Rest Position (*see* p. 81).

Watchpoint
Maintain a gentle engagement to your centre throughout to avoid the lower back becoming compressed.

HIP HINGE/ROLLING CAT
Stage 3

This is a wonderful stretch for the lumbar spine and to release tightness in your hips. If you have wrist pain either avoid this exercise, or place a cushion underneath the heel of your hands, or lengthen your hands slightly further away from you rather than directly under your shoulder joints.

- Begin in Four-point Kneeling (*see* p. 77). Lengthen your spine into neutral as you breathe in.
- Breathe out and hinge from the hip to send your bottom towards your heels. Keep the spine long, without tucking the tailbone underneath you.

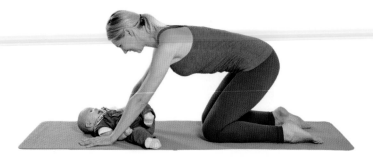

- Breathe in to push back to Four-point Kneeling, lengthening forwards over your hands to open at the hip joint. Repeat 5 times.

- Breathe out and curl the tailbone underneath you into a Cat, then release back towards your heels, maintaining this C-curve shape. This time feel the lumbar spine lengthening and stretching.

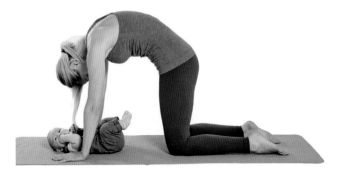

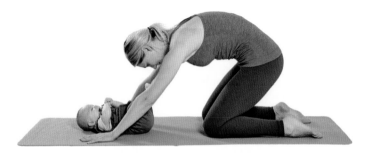

- Breathe in to push back to a neutral spine and release your weight forwards over your hands. Repeat 5 times.
- If you wish, you can create a 'rolling wave movement', leaning back in Cat then rolling forwards into an extension.

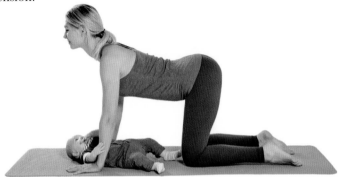

- Rest back into Rest Position (*see* p. 81).

THREE-MINUTE HEADSPACE MEDITATION

As a mum your time is more precious than ever before. You need some headspace to regulate your emotions and some breathing space for your body to soften, but don't want another thing to add to your to-do list. The Mindfulness-based Cognitive Therapy (MBCT) three-minute breathing space meditation is perfect.

You can find three minutes – notice whether you spend more than three minutes on social media, see if you can swap some of that to do this meditation instead, once a day. You can even just do the first part, in less than a minute – this is more than good enough if it's truly all you can find in your mothering day. Three deep breaths equals a meditation. A short meditation like this can serve to anchor you in a scattered day.

Step 1: Mind

Notice how things are in this moment, sit up tall and alert, like a meerkat. Close your eyes. Ask yourself, 'How am I feeling, right now?'

- What THOUGHTS are going through your mind? Try to acknowledge your thoughts as separate mental events, like clouds passing in the sky.
- What FEELINGS are here? Notice your feelings and emotions. Turn towards any discomfort or unpleasant feelings, acknowledging them, give them a hug.
- What BODY SENSATIONS can you feel? Pick up any sensations: tingling, tightness, bracing. Move in close to the sense of the breath in the abdomen … feeling the sensations of the abdomen wall expanding as the breath comes in … and falling back as the breath goes out. Follow the breath all the way in and all the way out, using the breathing to anchor yourself into the present.
- Now, try to describe what you notice – label your experience and invite them in (e.g. say in your mind, 'I feel a bit angry today' or 'Hello, self-critical thoughts').

Step 2: Heart

Redirect your attention to focus on the physical sensations of the breathing itself, within your ribcage, abdomen and heart centre.

Step 3: Body

Now expand your awareness around your breathing, to include a sense of your whole body: your posture, facial expression. If you become aware of any sensations of discomfort, tension, or resistance, breathe into them. Then breathe out from those sensations, softening and opening with the out-breath. Say to yourself, 'It's OK … whatever it is … Let me feel it.'

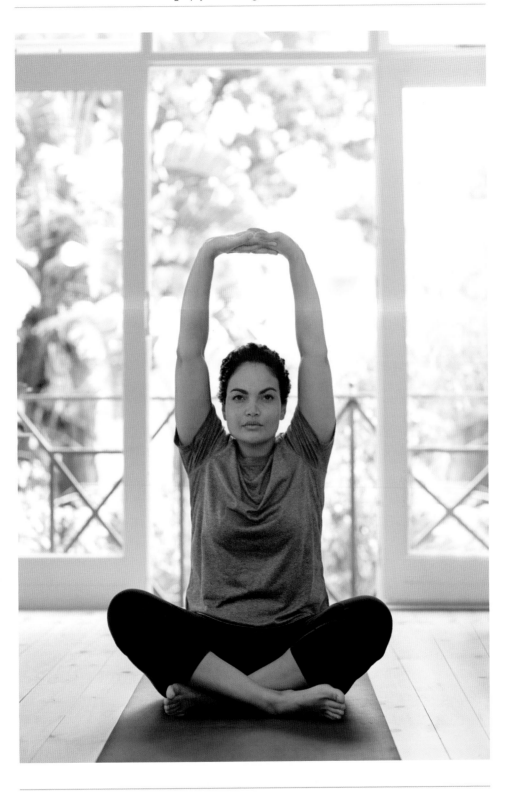

WORKOUTS FOR THE FIRST NINE MONTHS

5-minute workout	
Relaxation: Pelvic Floor: Pubic Bone Breathing 102	
Compass 75	
Spine Curls 82	
Roll-backs with Band 157	
Baby Cobra with Neck Roll and Twist 161	

10-minute workout			
Standing, Shoulder Stretch 67		Standing Wall Push Up 137	
Roll-downs Against the Wall 79		Squat with Arm Circle 154–5	
Mermaid with Twist 160			
Table Top Lift and Lower 159			
Dart 84			
Baby Cobra with Neck Roll and Twist 161			
Rest Position 81			

WORKOUTS FOR THE FIRST NINE MONTHS

20-minute workout

Three-minute Headspace Meditation   164

Pelvic Floor: Lift and Pulse 101	
Double Knee Folds 149	
Band Pull with Knee Drop 70	
Spine Curls 82	
Bridge with Double Knee Drop 83	
Ribcage Closure with Leg Extension 132	
Hip Rolls 87	
Hip Flexor Stretch 109	

20-minute workout cont.

Glute Stretch 111	
Curl-ups 147–8	
Back Release over Roller 150	
Oyster 72–3	
Prone Leg Circles 78	
Dart 84	
Hip Hinge/ Rolling Cat 162	
Legs Up the Wall 114	

Chapter 5

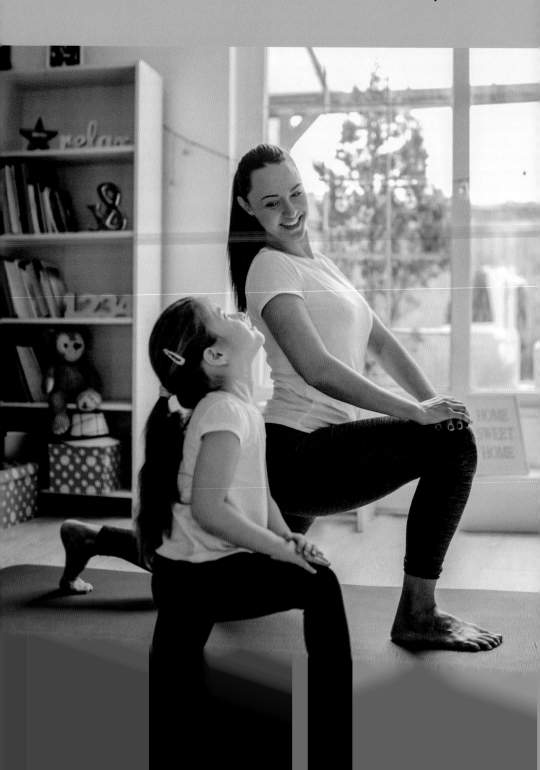

Year one and beyond

What is 'the postnatal period'?

It is not a small window of time that exists after you have a baby. It's not a finite period when you have temporarily become a mother. Often I'm asked by clients 'am I still postnatal, my baby's over a year?', or 'I had my baby two years ago so I'm not postnatal any more'. In my view, if you have ever had a baby, you are postnatal. For the rest of your life.

I think the word 'postnatal' is misunderstood – it's swept under the carpet, banished, humbled, belittled. We try to narrow it down to an arbitrary period of six weeks. Something to get through, to pass, to deal with and then move away from and 'get back to normal'.

But – you have *changed*. Your body, your heart, your mind has changed. Forever. You have experienced your matrescence. It's true that a very important and intense period of postpartum healing occurs in the few weeks and months after you have had your baby, when you're riding the hormonal and emotional rollercoaster and often in free fall, blindfolded. When that settles, you find an equilibrium. Often, the physical healing journey is ongoing – particularly if you've had a Caesarean birth or otherwise experienced physical or emotional trauma.

You may be craving getting back to 'regular life'. To have this postnatal period end and become 'normal'. Please be gentle with your new self. The postnatal period doesn't end just because you've stopped breastfeeding, gone back to work or once you fit into your pre-pregnancy jeans. You will be labelled by healthcare and most fitness professionals as 'no longer postnatal', but this undermines the fact that the physiological (and psychological) issues of pregnancy and birth have a long-term impact. Never allow yourself to be dismissed because you had your baby 'ages ago' but are still suffering from a weak core or pelvic floor issues. *Investigate* these things rather than wishing they would just somehow go away. You can always make yourself stronger.

The UK Chief Medical Officer Dame Sally Davies admitted in an article in the *Daily Mail* in 2018 that she still suffers from incontinence 20 years after having her babies. She is still, decades later, suffering from issues directly caused by giving birth, yet she wouldn't be classed as postnatal by the medical profession. I suspect that she's not alone in this experience. I met with Dame Sally in 2018 as part of campaign group the Pelvic Floor Patrol, to discuss with her how postnatal care could be improved and pelvic floor rehabilitation awareness. She told us that had she known about the benefits of physio and how regular pelvic floor exercises could impact on symptoms of pelvic floor dysfunction *this would have changed her life.*

That's your sign to *own your postnatal recovery.* You only get one life. Never stop checking in with your pelvic floor health, your mental health, your physical health, your emotional health. Be aware and curious. Never stop reaching out for information and guidance. Nothing breaks my heart more than hearing women say, 'of course my back and pelvic floor is buggered, I've had three children, it's too late now.' It's NOT too late. Don't settle for feeling like crap. Never belittle or ignore your needs. Never stop caring for yourself. You are always postnatal.

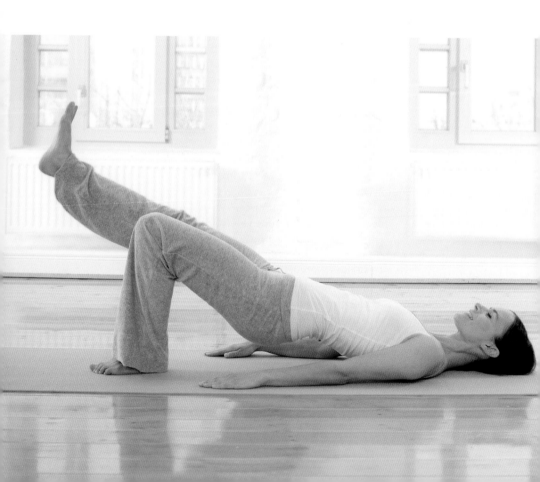

CURL-UP – ARM REACH AND KNEE DROP
Stage 3

I know that you want to feel that 'you're working' your abdominals and you want to get into 'regular exercise classes' again, or if you're a Pilates veteran, return to your beloved Pilates moves such as the 100 and Single Leg Stretch etc. Here is a Curl-up where you can truly challenge your pelvic stability and learn how to maintain a strong centre. If you see any doming or feel any pressure down onto your pelvic floor, you need to come back to your **Stage 1** exercises until you can control your intra-abdominal pressure. The pelvis needs to stay in neutral and supported by your muscles at all times. Perform slowly and with control. Release down if you feel any neck pain.

Remember the X Factor (*see* p. 70). Now find that connection even more consciously as you challenge your body with opposite arm and leg movements, while you are curled up.

- Begin in Relaxation Position (*see* p. 56), arms behind your head. Place the elbows into your peripheral vision, feel the shoulder blades widen on your back. Breathe in and lengthen.
- Breathe out, connect into your pelvic floor as you nod your chin towards your chest, curl your head and upper spine off the mat.

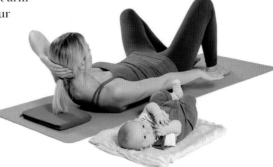

- Breathe in to lengthen and deepen your connection.
- Breathe out and release your right arm down by your side as you open your left knee out to the side.

- Breathe in to return to centre.
- Breathe out, then repeat on the other side.
- Repeat each side up to 5 times.
- Release back down and roll your head from side to side.

Watchpoints
The pelvis shouldn't rock and roll.
Keep breathing!

SPINE CURLS WITH CHICKEN WINGS
Stage 2

This is a lovely way of enhancing your pelvic floor awareness as gravity helps you to lift the muscles as your bottom lifts. It also opens your chest and makes you aware of your shoulder mechanics. Place a small ball between your knees for a bit more connection to your centre.

- Start in Relaxation Position (*see* p. 56).
- Breathe in. Lengthen your spine. Float your arms above your head and release them back behind you, resting them on the floor if you can, palms facing up.

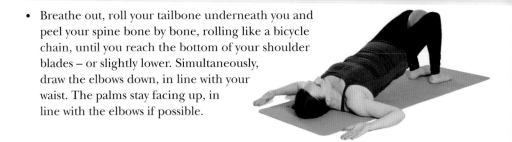

- Breathe out, roll your tailbone underneath you and peel your spine bone by bone, rolling like a bicycle chain, until you reach the bottom of your shoulder blades – or slightly lower. Simultaneously, draw the elbows down, in line with your waist. The palms stay facing up, in line with the elbows if possible.

- Breathe in, reach the arms back away behind you.

- Breathe out, soften your breastbone and release your spine back down, keeping your buttocks lifted and pelvis tucked under until you reach the floor.

- Breathe in to let go of any tension in the shoulders and hips, lowering your arms back down by your sides before repeating on the out-breath.

- Repeat up to 10 times.

Watchpoints

Remain open and relaxed across the shoulder blades.

Move with flow, coordinating the movement of your arms with your spine.

DUMB WAITER (WITH WEIGHTS, OPTIONAL)
Stage 2

This exercise strengthens your arms for holding your ever-growing baby, releases the front of your shoulders and opens your chest.

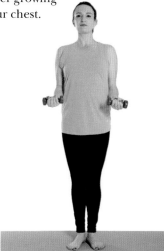

- Stand tall in Pilates Stance (*see* p. 88).
  Bend your elbows to approximately a right angle.
  Either: have your palms facing up, fingers
  lengthened and imagine you're holding a tray of
  drinks; or hold weights (or tins of beans) in your
  hands. Connect to your centre, lengthen your spine.

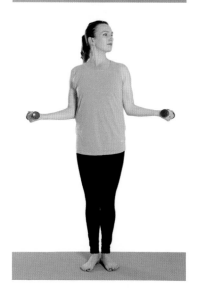

- Breathe in and rotate your arms outwards from
  the shoulder joint. Keep the elbows close to the
  waist, underneath the shoulders. The movement
  comes directly from the top of the shoulder, as if
  your shoulder is the hinge of a door opening.
  Look over one shoulder.

- Breathe out and return your arms and head
  to the start position.

- Repeat up to 10 times, to each side with
  your head.

- To add a challenge: bend your knees into a Plié
  (*see* p. 88) as you open the arms.

Watchpoint

Try to avoid pinching your shoulder blades together as this will encourage you to
arch your spine. Instead, imagine the collarbones and the shoulder blades soft
and open on the front and back of your body.

SIDE REACH ARM CIRCLE, INTO SIDE PLANK
Stage 3

A glorious stretch, for your side and for your hamstrings, this
challenges your balance, working shoulder and core muscles.
Take care if you have wrist/shoulder issues.

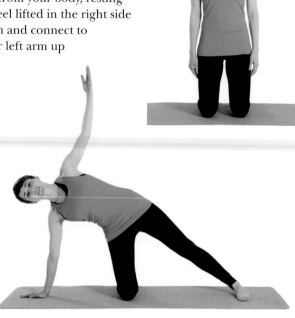

- From High Kneeling, reach your right arm down to
  the mat, placing your hand underneath your shoulder.
  Extend your left leg out away from your body, resting
  the whole foot on the floor. Feel lifted in the right side
  of your waist; the hips are high and connect to
  your core muscles. Reach your left arm up
  to the ceiling.

- Breathe in to reach the left arm over the head, then circle it
  down over the head, twisting the spine to reach it towards the
  floor, then up towards the hip and to the ceiling once more.
  Keep reaching into the foot
  of the top leg so there
  is a lovely stretch
  in the top side
  of the body.

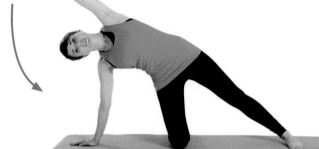

- Repeat 6–10 times.

- For more of a challenge, keep the left arm reaching up to the ceiling then use your core muscles strongly as you take the right leg to join the left leg, into full Side Plank.

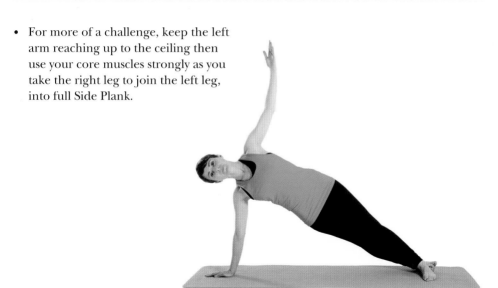

- To transition to the other side, place the left hand down to come into Four-point Kneeling (*see* p. 77) and push your bottom up into the air to come into Downward Dog. Take a few breaths here.

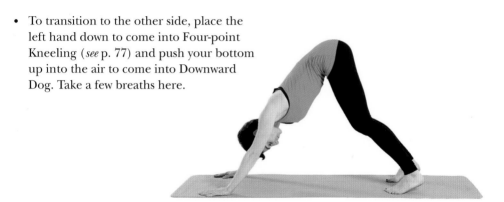

- Transition to the other side and repeat.

CAT WITH LEG EXTEND
Stage 3

This is a dynamic exercise that will challenge your balance and stability. You are moving swiftly between positions so you need to enlist your deep core, strengthening your arms, buttocks, tummy – a true whole-body exercise!

- Start in Four-point Kneeling (*see* p. 77). Lengthen into your neutral spine and breathe in to prepare.

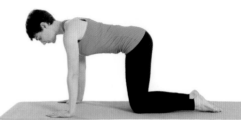

- As you breathe out, tuck your tailbone underneath and begin to curl into Cat (*see* p. 80). At the same time, bend your left knee in towards your centre, as you bend your right elbow in towards your left knee.

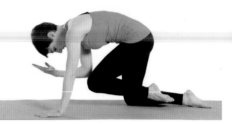

- Breathe in and reach the arm and leg away from each other, to body height – if this feels too dynamic, rest your hand and foot on the floor.

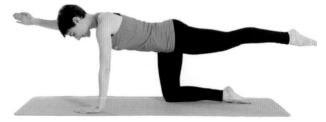

- Breathe out, curl your knee to your elbow and move into your Cat once more. Repeat the arm and leg extension on the same side, up to 10 times.
- Come back into Rest Position (*see* p. 81) if necessary, before repeating the exercise on the other side. Circle your wrists if they need a rest.

ELBOW TO KNEE
Stage 3

This is a challenging exercise that will get your blood flowing and give you an all-body workout. Take care to perform this mindfully if you are healing diastasis recti, as this exercise works your abdominals very strongly. Make sure you consciously connect to your pelvic floor and scoop your lower abdominals up and in, to encourage your deep corset of inner strength. You may need to build up strength for this one – start with only 2 or 3 repetitions and build up to 10.

- Start in Four-point Kneeling (*see* p. 77) and breathe in to lengthen the spine and prepare for movement.

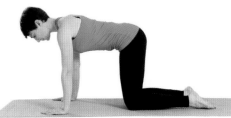

- As you breathe out, bend your left knee in and lift it to touch your left elbow. Your whole body will shift its weight forwards over your hands.

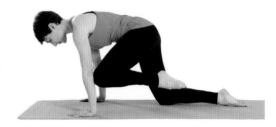

- Breathe in to straighten the left leg and reach it back in line with the body. Your weight will shift slightly back. Keep the spine long and supported.

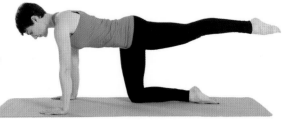

- Repeat up to 10 times, then release back into Rest Position (*see* p. 81) before repeating on the other side.

Watchpoint
Keep your leg at hip height as you reach it away, to make sure the spine stays lengthened, not arching.

LUNGE AND BALANCE
Stage 3

The great thing about doing standing work is that you can easily transfer the feeling into your daily life with your small people, and it's a good way of working your pelvic floor awareness and balance. If you're feeling scattered and overwhelmed, focusing on your balance is a wonderful means of calming the mind. Plus, it makes you feel strong, which can be emotionally as well as physically uplifting. You can keep the arms by your side if raising them is too challenging.

- Begin in standing. Step your right leg back behind you, keeping your feet hip-width apart and your pelvis square. Bend the right leg softly, raising the heel. Lengthen tall through the spine.

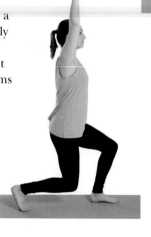

- Bend your left leg to lower into a Lunge. Lower your torso directly down, staying upright through the crown of your head, without tipping forwards. Raise your arms above your head.

- Breathing out, stand back up tall and fold the right leg in, bringing the right knee in line with your hip. Press the arms back slightly behind you, to feel the tricep muscles active. Take care not to arch the back.

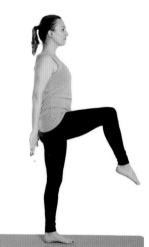

- Release back down into a Lunge, raising the arms and bending both legs.
- Repeat in the same direction up to 10 times, then change sides.

Watchpoint

If lifting the leg throws off your balance, just stay with a Lunge up and down, until you have the strength to balance as well.

JUICY HIPS
Stage 2

This is technically a yoga Pigeon pose, but I'm stealing it and changing its name. We hold a lot of tension in our pelvic area, particularly when children are a factor. A hip stretch releases tension and connects you to your centre, unlocking any tightness that might be affecting your lower back and pelvic floor. 'Hips don't lie', as Shakira said.

- Start in Four-point Kneeling (*see* p. 77). Fold your right knee in to rest by your right hand. Allow the foot to release down towards your left hip. Next, lengthen your left leg back behind you, extending it away along the floor.

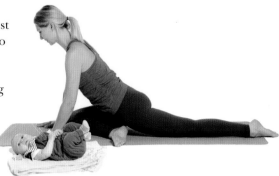

- Lift up through your centre and send your left leg away to stretch into the front of the hip.

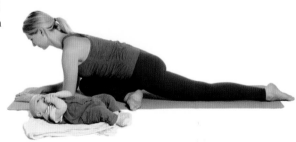

- Breathing long and deep, slowly release your torso forwards and down towards the mat.

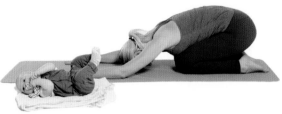

- Breathe deeply into the stretch, for as long as you feel comfortable, then carefully release yourself back up and change sides.
- Lower yourself back into Rest Position (*see* p. 81) to finish.

POSTNATAL MUM BUM LIFT
Stage 3

This is a great toner for your bum and inner thighs, mobilising your lower spine and pelvis. It's deceptively challenging – if you do this every day you'll have buns of steel in no time. You're lying down, so follow it with Legs Up the Wall (*see* p. 114). It can also be done with a toddler sitting on your chest, or for added load, draped over your shins...

- Lie on a mat, next to the wall. Shuffle your bum closer to the wall so that you can place your feet flat against the wall, with your knees at a right angle, feet slightly apart. Place a cushion or small ball between your knees. Release your arms down by your side.
- Breathe in to lengthen through the spine.

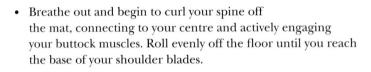

- Breathe out and begin to curl your spine off the mat, connecting to your centre and actively engaging your buttock muscles. Roll evenly off the floor until you reach the base of your shoulder blades.

- Breathe normally and, keeping your bum lifted, squeeze your inner thighs and buttocks. Then release. Then squeeze. Begin by pulsing slowly and build up to rapid quick pulses. You're not *moving* your bum or lifting it, just squeezing your muscles, which will enable a slight lift and release motion. Build up to 20, then 30.

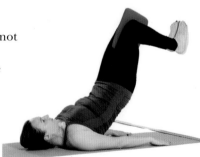

- On an out-breath, release your spine down, lowering bone by bone.

MAKE IT EASIER

If this is too much of a challenge or causes any discomfort in your neck, spine or pelvic floor, you can instead place your bum on the small ball, as for Compass on the ball (*see* p. 75–6), and, resting your bum down, gently bounce up and down on the ball up to 30 times.

DEAD BUG
Stage 3

This is a great challenge for the abdominal muscles – make sure you focus on stability, not allowing the back to arch or the pelvis to tip towards your heels. You can do this with a small ball underneath your pelvis for added challenge.

- Lying in Relaxation Position (*see* p 56), lengthen your arms up above your shoulders, palms facing forward. Float your first knee, followed by your second, into Double Knee Fold (*see* p 149). Your pelvis and spine are in neutral.

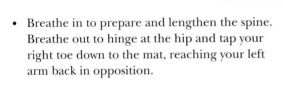

- Breathe in to prepare and lengthen the spine. Breathe out to hinge at the hip and tap your right toe down to the mat, reaching your left arm back in opposition.

- Breathe in to return to centre.
- Breathe out and release the opposite arm and leg on the other side.
- Be really conscious of your torso – whether you're hitching and dipping your pelvis, whether you're arching your back. Stay steady and strong.
- Repeat 8 times on each side, then bring your knees into your chest to finish.

Watchpoints

Make sure your *knee* isn't bending to bring your lower leg to the mat – hinge from the hip, the angle of the knee doesn't change.

Imagine you're dipping your toe onto water then bringing back up.

PELVIC FLOOR MEDITATION

This meditation cultivates a mindful awareness of our body. Tuning into our sensations at rest enables you to be able to connect to them actively in movement.

You can do this meditation sitting or lying down, whichever you feel more comfortable. It can take 2 minutes or up to 20, you choose.

- Soften your gaze inwards, closing your eyes. Tune in gently to the sensations of your breath, the rise and fall of your lower belly as you breathe in and out.
- Visualise a diamond shape filling in the space between your tailbone, your sit bones and your pubic bone. As you breathe in, imagine this diamond shape widening and opening.
- As you breathe out, imagine that it draws in and closes, almost like a camera shutter.
- Continue to breathe and simply notice that shape in your mind's eye. If your mind wanders, that's completely normal so don't berate yourself, simply notice and come back to the visual shape of the diamond and the sensations of your breath in the body.
- Then, begin to actively draw the shape up into your centre on your out-breath, actively recruiting the deep inner muscles.
- Breathe in to let them fully go.

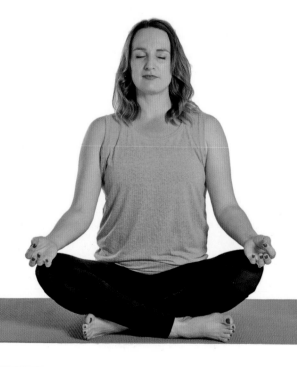

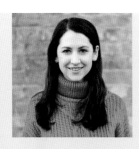

EXPERT ADVICE

Clare Bourne, mum of one, is a specialist women's health physiotherapist, based in London. Her particular area of interest is postnatal recovery and rehabilitation, working with women whatever their pregnancy and birth experience to achieve their goals. Her passion is that women feel heard, understood, educated and empowered at a time that can feel daunting and lonely. You can follow her on Instragram: @clarebournephysio.

I learned first hand the impact of pregnancy and childbirth on the body when I had my daughter. Even though I knew the theory up until this point, living it was a whole other story. On paper, I had a low-risk, uncomplicated pregnancy with a pretty textbook natural birth – HOWEVER, this has not meant that I got away without any pelvic floor dysfunction, or the need for my own physiotherapy and pelvic floor rehabilitation. Let's be honest – whatever the exit route of your baby, birth is intense.

For so many of us, pelvic floor exercises are the things we mean to do more of, tried but just got bored of, or just couldn't work out what we were meant to do so just stopped. I always say to women – 'I talk about them all day and I still forget to do them!' – so we all live in reality, it's not always easy to fit them in. That is why I love and encourage women to do Pilates as it is far more interesting than just sitting there doing your pelvic floor on its own – now don't get me wrong, there is definitely a place for that, especially in the early postnatal period. However, for me there was definitely a point when I just felt I was making no further progress with my pelvic floor strength. At this point I did more and more Pilates, and learning to use my pelvic floor again during movement, which I could put into everyday life, made a MASSIVE difference.

Feeling lost when we are postnatal is normal; most women I meet are not sure what to do, where to turn or how to get back to their 'normal'. The honest answer is everyone's journey is different, but having a comprehensive assessment like a Postnatal Body Check that we provide at SIX Physio, or a Mummy MOT, which is carried out by practitioners all over the country, is a great place to start. If you are going to invest in anything postnatal – this is it. However, your GP can also refer you to a women's health physiotherapist if you ask.

My top postnatal tips:

- Posture is one of the most important things postnatally, so definitely follow the guidance in this book closely and work on your posture in all positions; your body will thank you.

- Sex (that's right, I said it): this can be painful for a number of reasons, whether you've had a vaginal or abdominal birth, and is called dyspareunia. This is due to hormonal changes during breastfeeding that make the vaginal tissues dryer, or due to scar tissue either within the pelvic floor, or from the Caesarean. Scar massage and the use of lubrication can really help, but don't suffer in silence, you can get help; it often needs a bit more help than 'having a glass of wine or two to relax you' – as too many of my clients have been told!

- Don't rush: in the long run you will feel and look better if you take it slowly and get the deeper core muscles working gradually. I see a lot of women who have worked really hard at exercise but their tummy still doesn't 'look right' to them – and most of the time this is because they are not recruiting their muscles correctly. Follow Anya's step-by-step stages and you will be well on your way.

WORKOUTS FOR LIFE

5-minute workout

Windscreen Wiper Legs 105	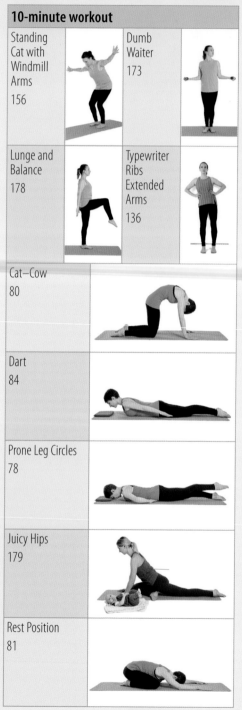
Bridge with Double Knee Drop 83	
Curl-up – Arm Reach and Knee Drop 171	
Side Reach Arm Circle, into Side Plank 174–5	
Relaxation Position 56	

10-minute workout

Standing Cat with Windmill Arms 156		Dumb Waiter 173	
Lunge and Balance 178		Typewriter Ribs Extended Arms 136	
Cat–Cow 80			
Dart 84			
Prone Leg Circles 78			
Juicy Hips 179			
Rest Position 81			

WORKOUTS FOR LIFE

20-minute workout		20-minute workout cont.	
Spine Curls with Chicken Wings 172		Table Top Lift and Lower 159	
Hip Rolls 87		Elbow to Knee 177	
Double Knee Fold 149		Stretch and relaxation sequence 109	
Dead bug 181		Postnatal Mum Bum Lift 180	
Oyster 72–3		Legs Up the Wall 114	
Side Reach Arm Circle, into Side Plank 174–5		Pelvic Floor Meditation 182	

Acknowledgements

Many thanks to all my Pilates clients over the past 10-plus years, who have provided inspiration and feedback for exercises included throughout the book. And to all the lovely babies I've held, jiggled and juggled over the years while giving their mums space to exercise.

Thank you so much to Emma Brockwell, women's health physiotherapist, Founding Member of Pelvic Roar (@pelvicroar) and Mummy MOT practitioner, who read the manuscript for accuracy and offered me her feedback and honest thoughts, and for being an outstanding pelvic floor/postnatal health guru and women's health cheerleader. Thanks also to Clare Bourne, physiotherapist at Six Physio and for @mummytribe who double-checked the manuscript just to be extra sure. You're both busy mums and I'm forever indebted to you for taking the time. Thank you to Kate Fry, who is a women's health physio and inspirational Pilates teacher, for your guidance and advice on this manuscript, and for your phenomenal breadth of knowledge around diastasis recti (and for correcting my floating ribcage!).

So many inspirations and sources of pelvic floor and diastasis recti advice and information are relevant in my continued professional development as a Pilates teacher, but in particular: Maeve Whelan from Pelvic Physiotherapy and Lynne Robinson at Body Control Pilates.

Huge thanks to Charlotte Croft and Sarah Skipper at Bloomsbury for making this passion project a reality. Thanks so much to my lovely models and mamas Denise, Simone and Gemma, not forgetting delicious baby Noah, for giving their time and movement for the book.

Thank you to my husband as always for putting up with being married to a writer. And my two crazy, wonderful boys Maurice and Freddie – you are the best and taught me everything I know on my continuing postnatal journey.

Resources

Suggested books

Bowman, Katy, *Diastasis Recti: the Whole-Body Solution to Abdominal Weakness and Separation* (Propriometrics Press, 2016)

Chatterjee, Rangan, *The 4 Pillar Plan: How to Relax, Eat, Move and Sleep Your Way to a Longer, Healthier Life* (Penguin Life, 2017)

Franklin, Eric, *Pelvic Power: Mind/Body Exercises for Strength, Flexibility, Posture and Balance for Men and Women* (Princeton Book Company, 2003)

Hands, Beccy and Alexis Stickland, *The Little Book of Self-care for New Mums* (Vermillion, 2018)

Hayes, Anya and Dr Rachel Andrew, *The Supermum Myth: Overcome anxiety, ditch guilt and embrace imperfection* (White Ladder, 2017)

Johnson, Kimberly Ann, *The Fourth Trimester: A Postpartum Guide to Healing Your Body, Balancing Your Emotions, and Restoring Your Vitality* (Shambala, 2017)

Kalinik, Eve, *Be Good to Your Gut* (Piatkus, 2017)

Myers, Thomas, *Anatomy Trains* (Elsevier, 2013)

Neufeld, Suzannah, *Awake at 3am.: Yoga Therapy for Anxiety and Depression in Pregnancy and Early Motherhood* (Parallax Press, 2018)

Ou, Heng, *The First Forty Days: The Essential Art of Nourishing the New Mother* (Abrams Books, 2016)

Panagos, Angelique, *The Balance Plan: Six Steps to Optimize Your Hormonal Health* (Aster, 2017)

Serrallach, Oscar, *The Postnatal Depletion Cure: A Complete Guide to Rebuilding Your Health and Reclaiming Your Energy for Mothers of Newborns, Toddlers and Young Children* (Sphere, 2018)

Stadlen, Naomi, *What Mothers Do, Especially When it Looks Like Nothing* (Piatkus, 2012)

Articles, TED talks

Benjamin, D.R., van de Water, A.T. and Peiris, C.L. (2014). 'Effects of exercise on diastasis of the rectus abdominis muscle in the antenatal and postnatal periods: a systematic review', *Physiotherapy*, 100(1), 1–8

Gilleard, W.L. and Brown, J.M.M. *Structure and function of the abdominal muscles in primigravida during pregnancy and the immediate post-birth period* (Southern Cross University ePublications@SCU, 1996)

Fernandes da Mota, P., Pascoal, A., Carita, A. and Bø, K. (2015). 'Prevalence and risk factors of diastasis recti abdominis from late pregnancy to 6 months postpartum, and relationship with limbo-pelvic pain', *Musculoskeletal Science & Practice*, 20(1), 200–205. DOI: http://dx.doi.org/10.1016/j.math.2014.09.002

Swift, S.E., Tate, S.B. and Nicholas, J. (2003). 'Correlation of symptoms with degree of pelvic organ support in a general population of women: what is pelvic organ prolapse?' *American Journal of Obstetrics and Gynaecology*, 189(2), 372–377

Pilates relating to incontinence symptoms https://bmcwomenshealth.biomedcentral.com/articles/10.1186/s12905-017-0503-y

NICE 2019 Guidelines for the treatment of Urinary Incontinence and Pelvic Organ Prolapse https://www.nice.org.uk/guidance/NG123

Returning to running postnatal – guideline for medical, health and fitness professionals managing this population https://www.researchgate.net/publication/331608702_Returning_to_running_postnatal_-_guideline_for_medical_health_and_fitness_professionals_managing_this_population

Dr Alexandra Sack's TED: A new way to think about the transition to motherhood www.ted.com/talks/alexandra_sacks_a_new_way_to_think_about_the_transition_to_motherhood

Useful websites

Bladder & Bowel Community
www.bladderandbowel.org

Breastfeeding support
www.vanessachristie.com

www.breastfeedingnetwork.org.uk/breastfeeding-support/

Cranial osteopathy
https://breastfeeding.support/cranial-osteopathy-or-craniosacral-therapy/

Chartered Society of Physiotherapy
www.csp.org.uk

Diane Lee: for information on pelvic floor health and recovery
www.dianeleephysio.com
https://dianeleephysio.com/education/diastasis-rectus-abdominis-postpartum-health

Holistic Core Restore®
www.holisticcorerestore.com

Julie Wiebe: Women's health physio specialising in pelvic floor recovery and Piston Breath
www.juliewiebept.com

Matrescence and transition to motherhood
www.matrescence.com

Make Birth Better – advice, support and information for birth trauma sufferers
www.makebirthbetter.org

Mummy MOT – postnatal health check covering pelvic floor and diastasis recti
http://themummymot.com/about/

NCT Hidden Half
www.nct.org.uk/hidden-half

NHS Start4Life Breastfeeding advice
https://www.nhs.uk/start4life/baby/breastfeeding/breastfeeding-challenges/mastitis/

Pelvic Obstetric & Gynaecological Physiotherapy (formerly Association of Chartered Physiotherapists in Women's Health)
http://pogp.csp.org.uk

Pelvic physiotherapy
www.pelvicphysiotherapy.com

Pelvic girdle pain charity support group
www.pelvicpartnership.org.uk

Pelvic Roar – information about pelvic health and women's health physiotherapy
www.pelvicroar.org

About the Author

Anya is a Pilates instructor, Mindfulness-Based Cognitive Therapy (MBCT) teacher and author specialising in pre and postnatal vitality and self-compassion. Anya is on a mission to empower women with the tools to navigate the landscape of modern motherhood with pelvic floor and sanity intact. Anya blogs at motherswellnesstoolkit. wordpress.com where you'll find self-care tools to help you build physical and mental resilience. Join the conversation on Instagram @mothers.wellness.toolkit. She has two boys, Maurice, 7, and Freddie, 4.

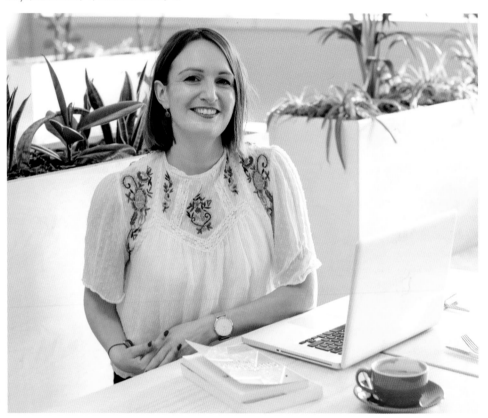

Index

Entries in *italics* are exercises.

abdominal massage 124–5
abdominal massage 127
abdominal muscles 44–7
abdominal overhang 126
adductor stretch 111
adhesions 125
alignment 11, 42, 52, 55
anxiety, after pregnancy 26, 32
author's postnatal experience 22–5
awareness stage 27, 44

'baby blues' 33
baby cobra with neck roll and twist 161
back release over roller 150
back stretch using the wall/buggy 65
backs, and lifting 53–4
band pull with knee drop 69, 70
band raise 134
bladders 42, 43, 44, 62
   see also incontinence
bodily changes
   after pregnancy 31–2, 33–7
   during birth 38–48
   during pregnancy 31
boobs, after pregnancy 25
'bounce back', pressure to 47
breastfeeding 103–8
breathing 11–12, 42, 58–9
bridge with double knee drop 83
build on it stage 28, 44

Caesarean sections 119–22
   exercises 127–39
   operations 122–3
   post-Caesarean healing 123–6
   workouts 140–1
cat with leg extend 176
cat-cow 80
centring 10–11, 60–2
centring in four-point kneeling 77

chalk circles 85–6
collagen 128
compass 75–6
concentration 10
coordination 12
curl-ups 147–8
curl-ups with leg slide 148
curl-up–arm reach and knee drop 171

dart 84
dead bug 181
depletion, postnatal 19–20, 21, 32, 143, 145
diastasis recti (DR) 26, 35, 44–7, 177
   REC check 49
   six-week check 95
diet 18–19
double knee folds 149
dumb waiter 173

elbow to knee 177
episiotomy 96, 97
equipment 15

fatigue 26–7
   see also rest
feet 51
flowing movements 12
foundations stage 28, 44
fourth trimester
   and birth trauma 95
   emotional health 91–2
   exercises 99–105, 108–14
   postnatal body 92–3, 96–8
   posture for feeding 107
   six-week check 93–5
   workouts 116–17

glute stretch 111

healing, postnatal 25–7

hip flexor bow and arrow 151
hip flexor stretch 109
hip flexor stretch with rotation and half snow angels 110
hip hinge/rolling cat 162–3
hip rolls 87
hormones 10, 33, 34, 35, 51, 95, 144
hypertonicity 43–4

incontinence, urinary 26, 33, 36, 40

Johnson, Kimberly Ann 32
juicy hips 179

knee drops 69

lateral flexion 88–9
leg slides 68
legs up the wall 114
lifting 53–4
lunge and balance 178

matrescence 31
meditations 21
    three-minute headspace 164
mental health 7, 10, 13, 17, 164, 170
    anxiety and emotions 26, 33
    fourth trimester 91–2
    postnatal depression (PND) 20–2
    see also wellbeing
mermaid with twist 160
modified push-up 138–9
Myers, Thomas 129
Myofascial lines 129

'naval to spine' 11
neck stretch and release 108
neutral pelvis and spine 55, 57
nine months out period 143–5
    posture 146
    strengthening exercises 147–64
    three-minute headspace meditation 164
    workouts 166–7

oyster 72–3

pelvic elevator 100
pelvic floor: lift and pulse 101
pelvic floor: pubic bone breathing 102
pelvic floor 39–42, 170
    dysfunction 26, 28, 40, 43, 49
    exercises 40–2
    healing 98
    restoration 44
    and the six-week check 94–5
    stability exercises 68–78
pelvic floor connection 62
pelvic floor meditation 182
pelvic organ prolapse (POP) 42, 63
pelvic tilts 57
pelvic tilts push with feet 129
pelvis 38–9, 55
    see also pelvic floor
perineum 40, 96–8
physios 35, 36
    nine months out period 146
Pilates method (defined) 9
piston breath 59
plantar fasciitis 51
Pliés with side reach 88
Post-traumatic Stress Disorder (PTSD) 95
postnatal depression (PND) 20–2
postnatal mum bum lift 180
postnatal period, defined 169–70
posture 52–4, 183
    for breastfeeding 107
    nine months out period 146
prone leg circles 78

Raphael, Dana 31
REC check 49
rehydration 17
relaxation 10
relaxation position 56
relaxation sequence 109–14
rest 17
    see also fatigue
rest position 81
revitalisation 18
ribcage 50
ribcage closure 74
ribcage closure with leg extension 132

roll-backs with band 157–8
roll-downs against the wall 79

Sacks, Alexandra 31
scarf breathing 58
scars 25
　　Caesarean 127
seated pelvic roll-back 113
self-care pillars 17–18
Serrallach, Oscar 32
sex, postnatal 183
shoulder drops, fly breaths 130
shoulder stretch 66
shoulder stretch against the wall 67
side reach arm circle, into side plank 174–5
side-lying ball roll 112
side-lying elbow to knee 152–3
single knee folds with pelvic floor work 71–2
sitting cross-legged roll forward 135
six-week check 93–5
sniff, flop, drop 99
spine
　　extension 84
　　flexion 79
　　movements of the 79–83
　　neutral 55
　　rotation 85–7
spine curls 15, 82
spine curls with chicken wings 172

squat with arm circle 154–5
stamina 13
standing cat with windmill arms 156
standing wall push-up 137
stretch marks 25
stretching sequence 109–14

table top leg extend 103
table top lift and lower 159
thigh stirs 104
traumatic birth 95
twisting spine curl 133
typewriter ribs extended arms 136

upright hip flexor side reach 89

wall posture check and side reach 64
wellbeing 7, 13, 18–19
　　see also mental health
Whelan, Maeve 99
Wiebe, Julie 59
windmill arms 131
windscreen wiper legs 105
workouts 13, 15
　　Caesarean recovery 140–1
　　first nine months 166–7
　　fourth trimester 116–17
　　for life 184–8
　　recovery 140–1